DM FRCS FRCOphth DO

Consultant Ophthalmologist,
University Hospital,
Nottingham UK

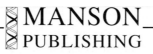

MANSON
PUBLISHING

A CIP catalogue record for this book is available from the British Library.

For full details of all Manson Publishing Ltd titles please write to
Manson Publishing Ltd, 73 Corringham Road, London NW11 7DL, UK.

Page layout: EDI Partnership
Project Management: John Ormiston
Colour reproduction: Tenon & Polert Colour Scanning Ltd, Hong Kong
Printed by: Grafos SA, Barcelona, Spain

CONTENTS

FOREWORD

Consideration of the full differential diagnosis is a discipline which lies at the heart of clinical practice. For beginners it does not become possible until they are familiar with the whole range of diseases that may cause the symptoms. For experienced practitioners it becomes all too easy to forget that rare disease should be considered. Therefore a disciplined approach to diagnosis must be used when the patient's condition is not immediately recognisable.

The clinical examination of the eye or its related structures often reveals the cause of the patient's complaint and it may be tempting to jump to the conclusion that a diagnosis has been reached. In reality the process is more complex. A careful history must be taken to determine the exact nature, severity and periodicity of the symptoms so that an exact match of symptoms to signs can be achieved. All too often hurried or incomplete analysis of the disturbance in vision or the nature of the discomfort leads to the wrong group of disorders being selected for differential consideration.

This book will guide all those who provide eye care, whatever their professional background.

Dr Jeffrey L Jay
Consultant Ophthalmologist,
Tennent Institute of Ophthalmology, Glasgow
and
President, Royal College of Ophthalmologists

PREFACE

To secure an accurate diagnosis in a patient presenting with a disorder of the visual system, the experienced doctor uses a strategy that proves or refutes specific diagnoses from his 'knowledge base'. This process commences during the history, with specific questions leading from the patient's presenting complaint. The examination is then performed to discover which of the differential diagnoses suggested by the history are present in that patient. This 'Baysean strategy' is very appropriate in ophthalmology where it is unusual to rely on special investigations to make the diagnosis. The strategy is helpful in busy clinics, casualty departments and in general practice as it is designed to make the diagnosis in the shortest (and therefore most efficient) time.

It must not be thought that this approach cuts corners compared with the traditional 'ask everything/examine everything' approach taught in many medical schools, although the latter is a valuable early learning tool. On the contrary, once the initial problem is diagnosed, time is then available to 'positively vet' for subtle physical signs which might be missed by other strategies.

Chapters 1 and 2 provide the grounding for the health care professional to make the diagnoses of conditions found in later chapters.

Chapters 3–10 each commence with a flow chart outlining the major conditions covered and a comment on the nature of symptoms necessary to be included in that chapter.

The order of chapters follows what I believe is a logical progression, though of course readers are free to use the material in any way they wish. As childhood problems usually form a discrete part of the specialty, I have chosen to place most of these in a separate chapter (3).

Where appropriate, guidance is given as to the frequency with which conditions present by the use of COMMON, UNCOMMON and RARE. Unless indicated, these refer to practice in the developed world with a population similar to that of the UK. Chapter 10 outlines some of the important ocular pathology seen in other areas of the world.

Conditions described in *italics* in the text have an accompanying illustration, and there are directions to another chapter where appropriate.

Stephen A. Vernon, 1998

Dedication

To my family for their patience and to all those from whom I have learnt over the years.

ACKNOWLEDGEMENTS

My thanks to Prof. Gordon Dutton for his permission to use the flow chart on nystagmus from our previous joint publication, *Passing Postgraduate Examinations in Ophthalmology* and to Miss A. Fiona Spencer for her comments on the penultimate draft.

CHAPTER I

ESSENTIALS OF ANATOMY AND PHYSIOLOGY

For the doctor aiming to make a diagnosis, principles are more important than detail, but a knowledge of what is normal must be obtained.

The visual system is made up of the ocular adnexa, the eyes and the brain. The ocular adnexa (bony orbit, lids, extraocular muscles, lacrimal gland and drainage apparatus, nerves and blood vessels) ensure the eyes have a suitable environment in which to provide the necessary sensory data for the brain to interpret.

Humans are binocular animals, with the ability to locate objects accurately in space (stereopsis). To do this each eye must provide the visual cortex with a clear image which can then be processed into a three-dimensional picture by the higher centres.

As with other primates, humans have both eyes facing forwards, although the apices of the **orbits** are directed medially (**1**). The optic nerve

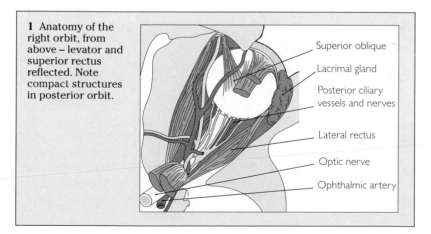

1 Anatomy of the right orbit, from above – levator and superior rectus reflected. Note compact structures in posterior orbit.

Superior oblique

Lacrimal gland

Posterior ciliary vessels and nerves

Lateral rectus

Optic nerve

Ophthalmic artery

and ophthalmic artery pass through the optic foramen and cranial nerves 3–6 and the superior ophthalmic vein pass through the superior orbital fissure. The origins of the rectus muscles and the levator palpebrae superioris surround the optic foramen, the muscle bellies of the recti projecting forwards to create an intraconal space. The **lacrimal gland** is sited in the superolateral aspect of the orbit and drains via 10–20 ductules into the superior fornix of the conjunctiva.

The **lids** prevent the cornea from drying by redistributing the tear film on blinking and by a physical barrier during sleep. In addition, they provide an outflow channel for excess tears by means of the punctae and canaliculi (**2**). Lid elevation is performed by the levator palpebrae superioris (3rd) with some assistance from the sympathetic system, whereas closure is effected by the orbicularis oculae (7th).

A normal **tear film** is essential for clear vision. The meibomian glands in the lids provide the outer lipid layer which prevents excessive evapo-

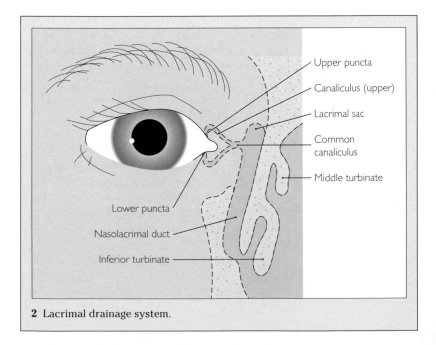

2 Lacrimal drainage system.

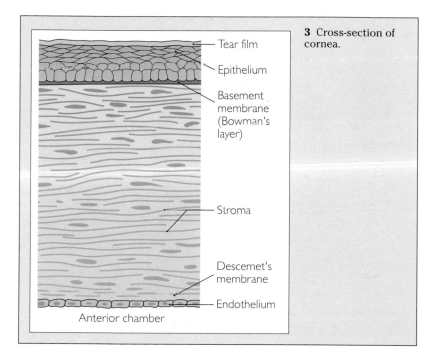

Tear film

Epithelium

Basement membrane (Bowman's layer)

Stroma

Descemet's membrane

Endothelium

Anterior chamber

3 Cross-section of cornea.

ration. The aqueous layer is separated from the epithelium of the cornea and conjunctiva by a mucous layer produced by the conjunctival goblet cells. Drying results in a disruption of the smooth refracting surface of the corneal epithelium, whereas inadequate drainage of excessive tears results in epiphora (overflow of tears onto the cheek). Both may cause varying degrees of disturbed sensation and vision.

The **cornea** provides two-thirds of the focusing power of the eye and must remain clear for a crisp retinal image (**3**). The epithelium is

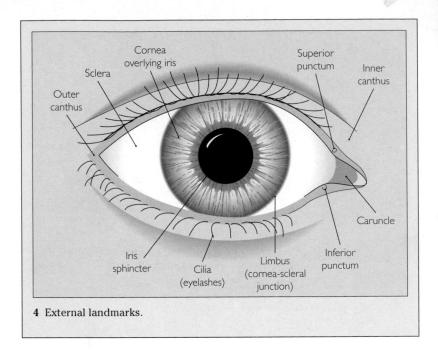

4 External landmarks.

continuous with that of the conjunctiva at the limbus (**4**) and is quickly regenerated following superficial trauma. The stroma, with its complex structure of accurately orientated collagen fibres, must be maintained in a relatively dehydrated state to allow light to pass through without reflection and dispersion. It is the corneal endothelium that is crucial in this process as it constantly pumps water from the stroma into the aqueous. An increase in water content, such as found resulting from very high intraocular pressure, leads to epithelial and then stromal clouding with reduced image quality. Similar effects on vision may be induced by scarring following certain inflammatory or traumatic processes.

The **lens** grows throughout life, adding extra fibres under its capsule and compressing the older fibres into its centre (nucleus). This results in a relative inability to change focus (accommodate) as one ages and the resulting optical effect is termed 'presbyopia'. A 'cataract' is defined as

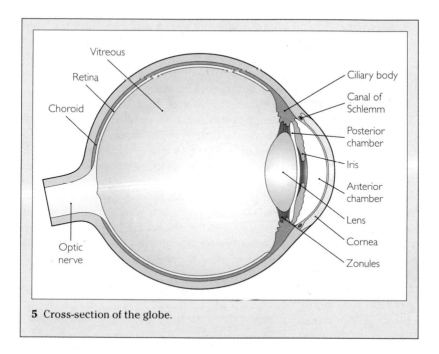

5 Cross-section of the globe.

any opacity in the lens (**5**). Cataracts may alter vision either by varying the focusing power of the lens, by reducing the overall image quality or, commonly, by a combination of both mechanisms.

The **iris** controls the amount of light entering the eye, preventing dazzle in bright conditions. Pupillary constriction is effected by a parasympathetic mechanism, whereas dilation is controlled by the sympathetic system. Accommodation, effected by the ciliary muscle, is linked to convergence of the eyes and pupillary constriction, all three mechanisms being mediated via the 3rd cranial nerve (oculomotor).

The **ciliary body** consists of the ciliary muscle, controlling accommodation via the zonules of Zinn and the lens, and the ciliary epithelium which secretes aqueous into the posterior chamber.

The **vitreous** is a gel containing 99% water, the remainder being mainly collagen and hyaluronic acid. Initially bonded to the lens and posterior retina in the child and young adult, the vitreous degenerates with age resulting in 'floaters' which are visible to most people under certain lighting conditions. A sudden separation of the body of the vitreous from the posterior retina (posterior vitreous detachment) can result in retinal tear formation which may lead to retinal detachment.

The **retina** contains the light-sensitive cells, rods and cones, and their supporting system of structural and information processing cells (**6**). The blood supply to the retina is via the central retinal artery, a branch of the ophthalmic, which enters the optic nerve 10 mm or so behind the globe. Its branches are end arteries, each supplying its own area of retina via a dense capillary network. Venous capillaries drain into branch retinal veins which run close to their supplying arterioles to form the central retinal vein on the optic nerve head. Around one million ganglion cell axons run on the retinal surface, curving towards the optic nerve head, which is situated 12–15° medial to the fovea. As eccentricity from the fovea increases, so the neuronal density decreases, thus the majority of the ganglion cells serve the central 30° of field.

Ganglion cell axons exit via the **optic nerve head** (optic disc), travel through the optic chiasm where nasal fibres (carrying temporal vision) decussate to form the optic tracts which synapse in the lateral geniculate body (LGB). From the LGB the optic radiations fan out to synapse with occipital cortex cells. Image information from the cortex is further processed by the visual association areas in the parietal lobes (**7**). Thus,

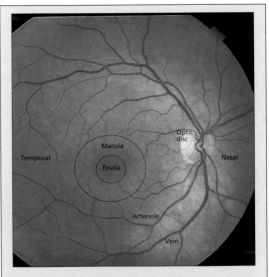

6 Retinal surface anatomy of a right eye.

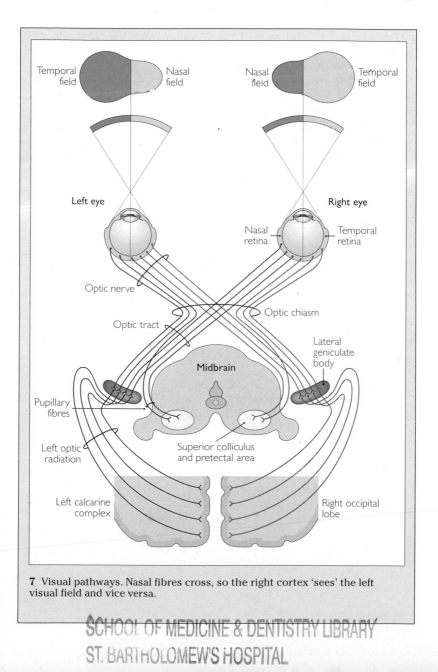

7 Visual pathways. Nasal fibres cross, so the right cortex 'sees' the left visual field and vice versa.

the left side of the brain 'sees' the right visual field (temporal right eye, nasal left eye) and vice versa. Many older patients lose one side of their vision from 'stroke' but errantly complain of a loss of vision in one eye.

Motor control of the eyes from the cortex enters the midbrain, which coordinates ocular movements using additional input from the cerebellum. Disruption of function at the midbrain results in specific syndromes affecting the movements of both eyes. Movements of an individual eye are effected by the 3rd, 4th and 6th cranial nerves operating through the extraocular muscles. The 4th nerve controls the superior oblique, the 6th the lateral rectus, and 3rd the remainder (medial rectus, inferior rectus, superior rectus and inferior oblique).

Most problems of ocular movement can be diagnosed by considering the primary actions of the extraocular muscles (see **19**).

CHAPTER 2

EXAMINATION OF THE VISUAL SYSTEM

Equipment

- A pen torch – providing a good bright directional light, preferably with a blue filter attachment (for use with fluorescein) (**8**).
- A low-powered magnifying loupe (×2 to ×3).
- A Snellen chart – for testing distance acuity (some are designed to be used at distances less than the standard 6 m for convenience).
- A reading test-type book – some pathologies may preferentially reduce reading ability in their early stages.
- A bright red target – for inter-eye colour comparison (some atropine bottle tops are ideal for this purpose).
- A 5-mm red pin, or pen top.
- An occluder – for determining the presence of squint.
- A pinhole – this can be incorporated in the occluder or made from cardboard.
- A good direct ophthalmoscope with halogen bulb.
- A slit lamp.

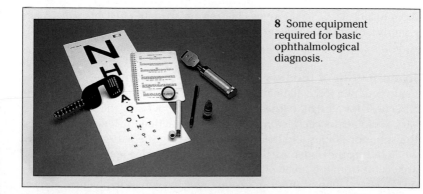

8 Some equipment required for basic ophthalmological diagnosis.

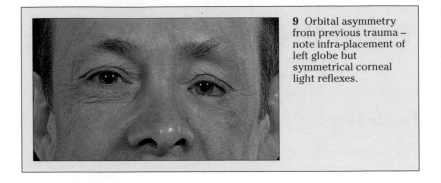

9 Orbital asymmetry from previous trauma – note infra-placement of left globe but symmetrical corneal light reflexes.

Basic techniques of ocular examination

General inspection

Before concentrating on the eyes, observe the patient for clues which may help your diagnosis. Look at the standard of dress and the colour of clothes worn – are they appropriate? Observe for any obvious limb weakness, and note the manner of speech.

Pay particular attention to the head and neck area. (Colour changes around the eyes can be easily missed when one has homed-in on one specific area.) Look for head turns and tilts, facial weakness, ptosis, *orbital asymmetry* (**9**) and proptosis. Proptosis is best excluded by viewing the seated patient from above and behind, while gently retracting the upper lids.

Shine your pen torch or ophthalmoscope beam at the patient, asking them to look at the light (young children are attracted to lights and usually comply). Check that the corneal light reflections are symmetrical (they should be just below and nasal to the centre of the pupil).

Examination of the lids and anterior segment

Using your pen torch, illuminate the eye from the lateral side at a 45° angle and check for a bright corneal reflection (reflex). Using the loupe if necessary, examine the *inferior fornix* by gently retracting the lower lid (**10**), and the superior limbus and conjunctiva by asking the patient to look down while raising the upper lid. Corneal oedema, scarring and vascularization are visible from this angle of illumination, particularly if the light is shone on the lateral limbus. Anterior chamber signs such as hyphaema, and iris

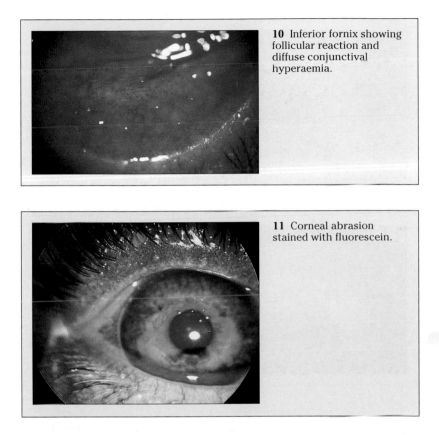

10 Inferior fornix showing follicular reaction and diffuse conjunctival hyperaemia.

11 Corneal abrasion stained with fluorescein.

and pupil details may also be observed. Move the torch to the equivalent position nasally and look again, as an altered angle of incident light may disclose further physical signs, especially of the cornea. Next, examine medial structures such as punctae and the caruncle.

The use of fluorescein and Rose Bengal

Examination following instillation of fluorescein is essential to exclude surface corneal pathology such as herpes simplex keratitis and *corneal abrasions* (11). A cobalt blue light is advised (staining defects green) but an ordinary pen torch light often shows epithelial defects which were unclear without the dye.

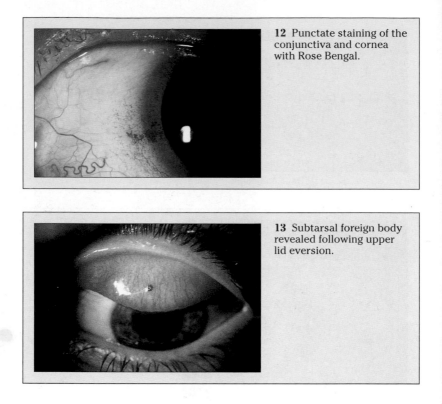

12 Punctate staining of the conjunctiva and cornea with Rose Bengal.

13 Subtarsal foreign body revealed following upper lid eversion.

If a diagnosis of 'dry eye' is being considered, Rose Bengal (available as single dose units) stains devitalized cells on the conjunctiva and cornea where drying is maximal. NOTE: Rose Bengal, unlike fluorescein, stings badly especially in dry eye states (**12**), and so a drop of a short-acting local anaesthetic is advisable prior to its instillation.

Everting the upper lid

This is best performed bimanually, with the forefinger and thumb of one hand pulling the lashes downwards while rolling the lid over a fulcrum (such as a glass rod or thin pencil) which has been positioned along the lid crease. This results in a view of the undersurface of the tarsal plate, a common site for *foreign bodies* (**13**).

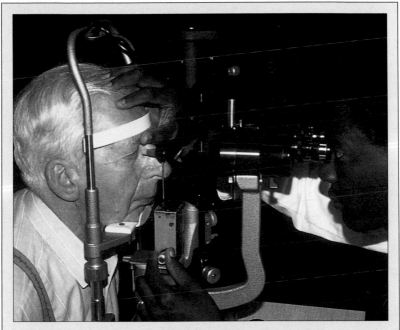

14 Goldmann applanation tonometry – it is advisable, if possible, not to hold the lids when performing pressure readings.

Estimation of intraocular pressure (IOP)

Although best tested with a *tonometer* (**14**), once experienced with the technique, one can detect an intraocular pressure (IOP) that is higher than 35 mmHg by digital tonometry. This is particularly useful in suspected acute angle closure glaucoma and advanced rubeotic glaucoma when the IOP may be 60 mmHg or more. Ask the patient to close both eyes and look down. Place the index finger of each hand gently on the upper lid with a separation of 1 cm centrally. Ballot the eye between the two fingers, judging the resistance to indentation. A feel for the normal obtained through practice allows significantly raised IOPs to be identified. This test must not be used if a very soft eye is suspected, such as after trauma or in the early postoperative period after intraocular surgery.

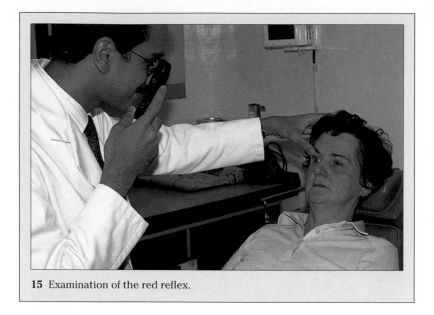

15 Examination of the red reflex.

Testing corneal sensation

Prior to any instillation of local anaesthetic, ask the patient to look into the distance and raise the eyebrows. From the side, gently touch the centre of the cornea with a wisp of cotton wool or tissue. A blink reflex should occur. Repeat on the other eye for a qualitative comparative test, making sure not to invoke a blink with a visual stimulus rather than a tactile one!

The ocular media

Lens pathology sufficient to cause symptoms is best diagnosed by *examining the red reflex* with an ophthalmoscope. To do this stand about 50 cm from the eye and view the eye through the sight hole of the instrument, ensuring that the iris is in focus (**15**). Any opacity is seen as a dark area in the red reflex. The relative position of opacities can be judged by viewing the red reflex from different angles. The more anterior an opacity, the more it appears to change its position with this manoeuvre. (Beware the patient with keratoconus – the distorted cornea creates a characteristic globule-shaped disturbance of the red reflex.)

Vitreous opacities, such as haemorrhage or cellular accumulation in posterior uveitis, create more blurred-edged obscurations in the reflex, or

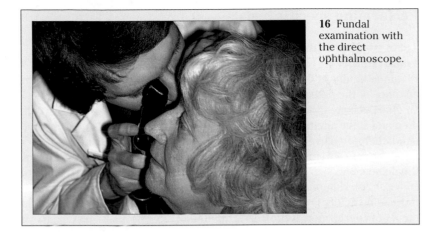

16 Fundal examination with the direct ophthalmoscope.

obliterate it altogether, particularly when viewing the reflex without pupillary dilation.

Fundoscopy

Having confirmed that the media are clear enough for fundal examination, a systematic approach is advisable when using the *direct ophthalmoscope*. The nearer you bring the ophthalmoscope to the eye the wider the field of view. Use your right eye to examine the patient's right eye, holding the 'scope in your right hand, and vice versa (**16**). Most patients find it reassuring if you gently place your other hand on their forehead, raising the upper eyelid if necessary.

Fundoscopy is best performed with a dilated pupil (0.5–1% tropicamide acts rapidly and wears off within 4–6 h). However, when dilation is contraindicated, the use of the small light aperture in a dim room may allow an adequate view of most of the retina. Examine the disc first, following the 'arrows' created by the bifurcations of the retinal vessels back to the disc if orientation is difficult. Next, follow the main four vessel pairs around the temporal and nasal arcades, scanning the nasal, superior, inferior and temporal retina (don't forget to ask the patient to look in the direction of the retina you want to see in order to improve your view of the periphery). Examine the posterior pole last, asking the patient to look directly into the light for a view of the fovea (dilated pupil essential).

Performing specific tests

Tests of visual function
Visual acuity
Distance acuity is usually measured with a *Snellen chart* – the correct distance of the patient from the chart must be maintained for the particular chart you are using. Remember to occlude carefully the other eye (children and some adults inadvertently peep between fingers of an 'occluding' hand; therefore cover the other eye yourself) (**17**). Test with suitable spectacles or contact lenses (beware the patient using 'reading' spectacles for the distance Snellen test!!). Use a pinhole (best diameter 1.5 mm) if acuity <6/6 (20/20). Number charts and pictographic charts for illiterates exist.

Reading acuity is tested with examples of *different sized print* (**18**) and the test is performed at the correct distance (35 cm) Again, test each eye separately with correction if required.

Colour comparison between the eyes
This test compares the depth of colour of a red target between the two eyes. Hold up the target in front of a white background and ask the patient to look at it with each eye in turn. A 'duller red' or 'orangey red' with one eye suggests optic nerve damage, despite good acuity in that eye.

Visual field testing by confrontation
The strategy suggested here is designed to detect large homonomous defects first, moving to more subtle defects later.

Sit 1 m in front of your patient. Ask him/her to look at your nose. Hold one finger of each hand in the superior quadrants. Make a small movement with one finger and ask the patient to point towards the movement. Repeat, moving the other finger, and again with both (testing for sensory inattention). Move your fingers to equivalent positions in the inferior field and repeat the above process. (If the patient does not see the small finger movements, gradually make them bigger until you are waving your hand.) A normal response effectively rules out significant homonomous hemianopias.

Now ask the patient to cover one eye (carefully!), and look at your nose again. Ask them if they can see the whole of your face clearly. This tests for central and paracentral defects – e.g. if with their left eye they cannot see your left eye, they have a left paracentral superonasal scotoma. Now continue with quadrant testing as described above and repeat for the other eye.

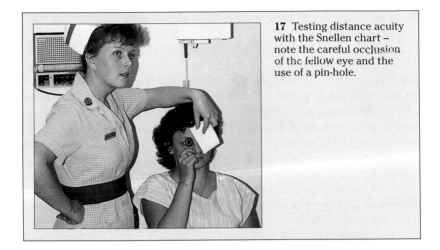

17 Testing distance acuity with the Snellen chart – note the careful occlusion of the fellow eye and the use of a pin-hole.

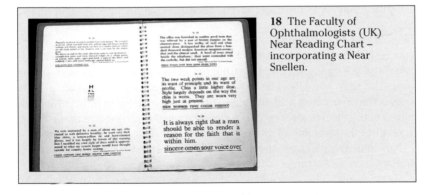

18 The Faculty of Ophthalmologists (UK) Near Reading Chart – incorporating a Near Snellen.

If no defect has been identified, perform 'the Union Jack' test. This test involves a systematic search for defects by screening along horizontal and vertical meridians (St. George's cross), followed by the diagonals (St. Andrew's cross) with a small target (preferably a 5 mm red pin). For each meridian, move the target from a non-seeing peripheral location to the centre, asking the patient to identify when they first perceive it and also whether it dims or disappears during its course towards fixation. This strategy eliminates all but the smallest scotomas. Examination for an enlarged blind spot (12–15° temporal to fixation) completes the field assessment.

Tests of muscle balance and ocular movement

The cover test

This test is to identify a manifest squint (strabismus). For adults and older children who will cooperate, ask the patient to fixate on a distance target (they should be wearing their distance correction). Cover their left eye while watching their right eye. If the latter moves at the moment of occlusion, the test is positive. An inward movement indicates a divergent and an outward movement a convergent squint. Repeat, covering the right eye this time, giving the patient time to refixate between tests. Vertical movements or a combination of horizontal and vertical can, of course, occur. Remember, for this test to be reliable, both eyes must have enough vision to be able to fixate on the target.

For young children, examine the position of the reflections induced from the corneae from an ophthalmoscope or pen torch. The physiological position is just nasal to the centre of the pupil. Asymmetry usually (but not always) indicates strabismus (this test simulates a distance target and therefore a small, interesting toy is used to stimulate accommodation). The cover test, using the torch/toy as the target, can be added to confirm a suspicion of squint.

The alternate cover test

This tests for a latent squint. If no abnormality was found on the cover test, cover the left eye again and wait 10 s before moving the cover rapidly to cover the right eye. Observe if the left eye moves to take up fixation. This reveals the presence of a latent squint, the degree of movement being an indication of the magnitude. The cover can be moved from one eye to the other to confirm the direction of movement and its size.

Now repeat both cover and alternate cover tests with the patient accommodating on a near target (at 35 cm).

Ocular movements

This test may be objective, the observer identifying a deficiency in the extent of ocular excursion(s), or subjective where the patient reports the presence of diplopia in various positions of gaze.

Start with the patient observing a pencil held vertically 1 m directly in front of him or her. Move it slowly to the left and then right to test the extremes of lateral gaze. On returning to the centre, position the pencil horizontally and test the extremes of elevation and depression in left and right gaze. The pencil thus makes a broad letter H in space. To confirm a suspicion of under/overaction of muscles, a cover test can be performed in any position of gaze. Finally, test convergence by moving a centrally located

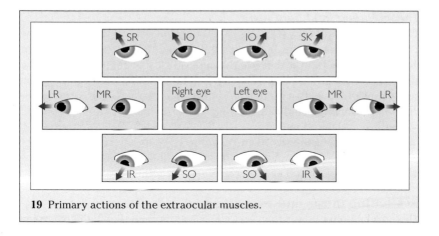

19 Primary actions of the extraocular muscles.

target towards the patient's nose. Remember the *primary actions of the extraocular muscles* and relate them to your findings (**19**).

Occasionally, it is helpful to test rapid saccadic movements (the above tests were using pursuit or tracking movements). Incomplete or recovering nerve palsies and midbrain syndromes may be accentuated by this strategy.

Testing the pupils

Abnormalities may be in size, shape or reaction. Always observe the size and shape of the pupils before testing their reactions. The reaction of the pupils are tested to a light and then to a accommodative target.

The pupil reactions to light may be abnormal in two ways, creating an afferent or an efferent defect. In an efferent defect there is an abnormality in the motor system of the reflex loop with a poor or absent constriction response of a pupil to a light shone in *either* eye *or* on accommodation. In an afferent defect, the sensory arm of the reflex loop is impaired, so reducing constriction of both pupils when a light is shone in the *affected* eye. In an absolute afferent defect (found in blind eyes), there is no pupillary constriction when a light is shone in the affected eye. More commonly, a relative afferent pupil defect is found and is best confirmed by the 'swinging flashlight test' (see below). If the afferent systems of both eyes are equally affected, as in retinitis pigmentosa, both pupils react sluggishly to light, but respond normally to accommodation. This is called 'light-near dissociation' and may be seen in any cause of severe bilateral global retinal or optic nerve disease. It is also seen in the dorsal midbrain syndrome due to damage to the pupilomotor fibres in the pretectal region.

The swinging flashlight test

This is a test to identify a relative afferent pupil defect (RAPD). With the patient viewing a distant target in subdued lighting, shine a bright light directly into the right eye. Move the light quickly to shine in the left eye and observe for any dilation of the left pupil (indicating a left RAPD). Then swing the light quickly back to shine in the right eye and again observe for dilation of the pupil (indicating a right RAPD). This test can be repeated to confirm initial findings.

If one pupil has already been shown to have an efferent pupil defect (e.g. dilated with tropicamide), the test can still be performed by observing only the pupil which has the capacity to react normally.

Evaluating ptosis and exophthalmos

The normal upper lid position (in Caucasians) is such that 2 mm of cornea is covered at 12 o'clock, and the lower lid just reaches the limbus at 6 o'clock. The lids remain in these positions when looking up or down as lid movements follow eye movements.

Ptosis indicates a relative lowering of the upper lid position. In exophthalmos (proptosis) and enophthalmos, the globe protrudes or is retro-placed such that both the upper and lower lid positions are usually abnormal. In lid retraction, an abnormally raised upper lid fails to lower in synchrony with the eye when looking down.

Proptosis can be axial or non-axial. In the former, such as occurs with a space-occupying lesion (SOL) inside the muscle cone, the eye protrudes directly forwards. In the latter, from an extraconal SOL, the globe is displaced forwards and away from the SOL. Measure the distance of the central cornea from the centre of the bridge of the nose with a ruler to detect lateral or medial displacement.

Proptosis can be measured with an exophthalmometer (Hertel test), or from the side using a plastic ruler placed carefully on the lateral margin of the bony orbit. A measured asymmetry of up to 2 mm in the anterior position of the cornea may be physiological.

Ptosis can be assessed with a ruler from the front, usually indirectly by comparison of central palpebral aperture widths (assure yourself that the lower lid position is normal and no proptosis or enophthalmos exists). Levator function is measured by asking the patient to look down, identifying the position of the upper lid margin on a ruler, and then again with the eye in maximum elevation. A finger or thumb on the eyebrow prevents the use of the occipitofrontalis and a false reading.

CHAPTER 3

THE CHILD WITH SUSPECTED EYE DISEASE

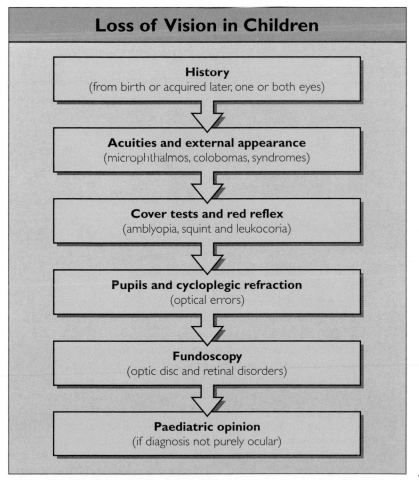

Loss of Vision in Children

History
(from birth or acquired later, one or both eyes)

Acuities and external appearance
(microphthalmos, colobomas, syndromes)

Cover tests and red reflex
(amblyopia, squint and leukocoria)

Pupils and cycloplegic refraction
(optical errors)

Fundoscopy
(optic disc and retinal disorders)

Paediatric opinion
(if diagnosis not purely ocular)

Strategy point – The History

An accurate history from the parents or carers before examination of the child defines which examination(s) is(are) necessary. In younger children the doctor is either screening for disease or symptoms and signs have alerted an adult's attention to the eyes. Older children usually present with symptoms only if they are perceived by the child to be outside their experience of normality. For example, the child developing myopia often, in the earlier stages, thinks that blurred distance vision is 'normal'. Only when they realise they are clearly different from their peers does presentation become more likely.

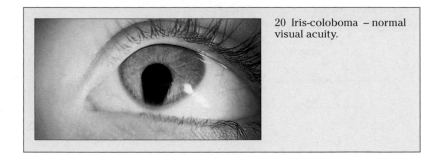

20 Iris-coloboma – normal visual acuity.

Screening the infant for ocular disease

All newly born children should be examined for congenital eye disease. Lids and anterior segments are examined with a pen torch for conditions such as *colobomas* (**20**), *aniridia* (**21**), microphthalmos and corneal clouding. *Congenital cataract* (**22**) is detected by examination of the red reflex (all RARE).

As ocular coordination does not stabilize until 3–4 months of age, variable squints are common in the newborn and if each eye appears normal, no action needs to be taken until after this age. Any squint persisting at 6 months of age requires referral to an ophthalmologist for full investigation.

Infants who are premature (<32 weeks' gestation) and/or light for dates (<1.5 kg) are referred to be screened for *retinopathy of prematurity* (**23**) by a paediatric ophthalmologist. This is most efficiently performed 6 weeks after birth and requires pupillary dilation and the use of an indirect ophthalmoscope.

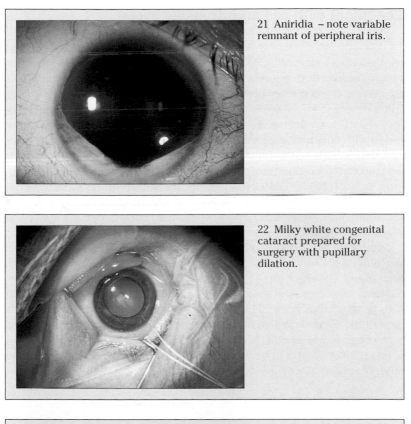

21 Aniridia – note variable remnant of peripheral iris.

22 Milky white congenital cataract prepared for surgery with pupillary dilation.

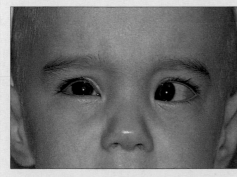

23 Retinopathy of prematurity inducing right microphthalmos and strabismus. The left eye is highly myopic but attained 6/9 (20/30) acuity when the child was older.

The infant with red and/or sticky eye(s)

An episode of conjunctivitis within one month of birth is termed *ophthalmia neonatorum* (RARE) (**24**). If silver nitrate has been used as prophylaxis against gonococcal ophthalmia, a chemical conjunctivitis is common in the first few days of life, but otherwise a child with swollen lids and a purulent discharge within the first week of life is treated as gonococcal until proved otherwise. Later onset at 5–14 days is more often associated with chlamydial infection.

A persistently or intermittently sticky eye(s) after one month of age is most likely to be due to a *congenital delay in the patency of the nasolacrimal duct* (**25**) (COMMON). Typically, the child requires bathing of the eye after each period of sleep, but the conjunctiva remains white (unless secondary infection occurs). Spontaneous resolution before the age of one year occurs in 95% of cases.

Symptoms and signs requiring re-evaluation are focal conjunctival injection and/or photophobia. Check for corneal foreign body, corneal ulceration (with fluorescein), and corneal clouding. Always consider *buphthalmos* (congenital glaucoma) (RARE) (**26**) in an infant or young child with photophobia, corneal clouding and epiphora – the eye also appears larger than normal. Benign *megalocornea* (**27**) needs to be differentiated from congenital glaucoma. In the latter, symmetrical, condition the cornea is larger than 13 mm in horizontal diameter at two years of age and is otherwise normal, as is the IOP and optic disc.

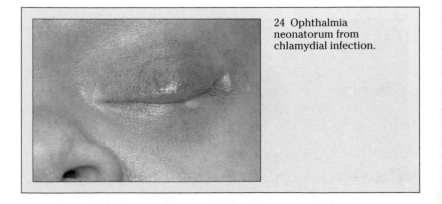

24 Ophthalmia neonatorum from chlamydial infection.

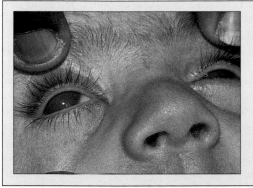

25 Delayed opening of the nasolacrimal duct – note white eye with excess mucus and increased tear film.

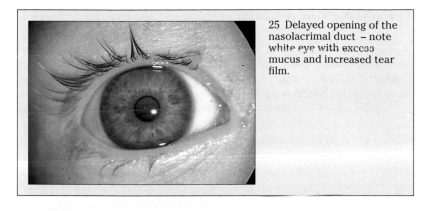

26 Bilateral congenital glaucoma (buphthalmos) with enlarged globes and corneal oedema.

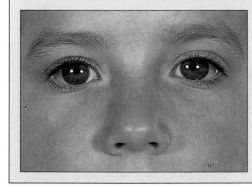
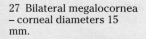

27 Bilateral megalocornea – corneal diameters 15 mm.

The older child with red and/or sticky eye(s)

In older children, acute sticky eyes which are sore and irritable are most likely to be infectious in origin with diffuse conjunctival injection (see Chapter 6).

Bacterial conjunctivitis (COMMON) (see **147**) is rapid in onset, almost invariably bilateral, and the purulent discharge renders the diagnosis simple, as does the response to treatment with broad-spectrum topical antibiotics such as chloramphenicol, sulfacetamide or gentamicin.

In *viral conjunctivitis* (COMMON) (**28**) there is often a history of upper respiratory tract infection in the child or the family, the discharge is watery rather than purulent, and follicles may be seen in the lower fornix after a few days (these are not seen in bacterial disease). Examine for a pre-auricular lymph node. Primary herpes simplex infection results in a vesicular rash often around the eyes, together with a bilateral conjunctivitis. A primary dendrite may occur. Adenovirus infection typically causes a very injected caruncle and may proceed to a secondary keratitis with photophobia.

A *follicular conjunctivitis* (see **151**), particularly if chronic, always prompts a search for *molluscum contagiosum* lesions (see **133**) along the eyelid margin.

In uniocular disease, also consider occult chalazia, corneal foreign body, herpes simplex keratitis and corneal ulceration.

Chronic itchy sticky eyes are typical of *allergic conjunctivitis* (see **149** and associated text). Hay fever conjunctivitis is found in older children (COMMON). The more serious *vernal catarrh* (RARE) is found in 5- to 15-year-olds. Itching, discharge and photophobia occurs together with giant papillae on the superior tarsal plates, seen after eversion of the upper lid (which may require local anaesthetic drops beforehand). *Limbal follicles* (**29**) may be seen at the superior limbus with punctate erosions in the upper half of the cornea, associated with pannus (a superficial ingrowth of vessels onto the cornea). In severe cases, sterile 'shield' ulcers may form on the cornea.

Although not necessarily red, a slowly growing *limbal dermoid* (RARE) requires recognition (**30**), together with a search for other features of Goldenhar's syndrome in which it is most commonly found.

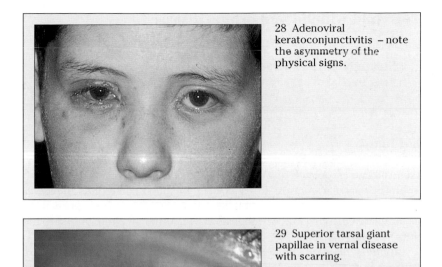

28 Adenoviral keratoconjunctivitis – note the asymmetry of the physical signs.

29 Superior tarsal giant papillae in vernal disease with scarring.

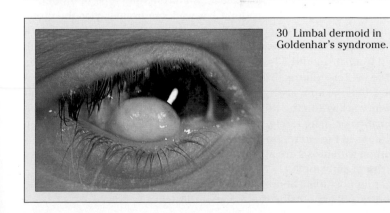

30 Limbal dermoid in Goldenhar's syndrome.

The child with lid and orbital disease

> ### Strategy point – History and external examination
> Look from above the forehead when suspecting proptosis.

Lid lumps

Lid lumps usually are acquired in the form of a *stye* or *chalazion* (COMMON) (see **169** and associated text). Large chalazia can produce a ptosis.

Of the vascular abnormalities (RARE), the most common is the *strawberry naevus* (haemangioma) which presents in the first few weeks of life as a rapidly enlarging purple/red lesion (**31**). Although often limited to the lid(s), orbital extension can occur.

Capillary haemangioma of the Sturge–Weber type (RARE) (**32**) are present from birth and easily diagnosed. It is associated with glaucoma which often commences in childhood, necessitating an examination under anaesthetic if in doubt. Orbital extension can occur.

Abnormalities of lid position (RARE)

In children, these are usually congenital or associated with acute inflammatory conditions. Congenital ptosis may be familial or associated with other abnormalities. Variable degrees of ptosis are seen and the child may use their occipitofrontalis to raise the lid on the least affected side, thus masking the bilaterality of the disease. An interesting type of uniocular congenital ptosis is the 'Marcus Gunn Jaw wink syndrome' when the ptotic lid twitches or rises during eating or sucking. A *congenital Horner's syndrome*, with a 2-mm ptosis and a relative meiosis (**33**), may be distinguished from an acquired lesion by the presence of heterochromia iridis (with the lighter-coloured iris on the affected side).

Other bulk lesions giving rise to ptosis include haemangiomas and *neurofibromas* within the lid (see **164**) and lacrimal gland swelling from inflammation or, more rarely, tumours. A typical 'S'-shaped swelling is seen with lesions in the lateral portion of the upper lid.

Children with ptosis are always referred to an ophthalmologist because of the risk of amblyopia.

Other lid positional abnormalities are usually associated with specific syndromes and are outside the scope of this text.

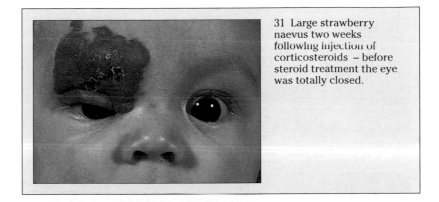

31 Large strawberry naevus two weeks following injection of corticosteroids – before steroid treatment the eye was totally closed.

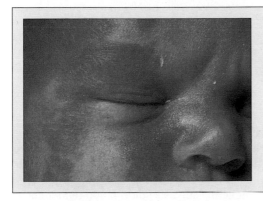

32 Sturge–Weber syndrome – port-wine stain – upper lid involvement increases the probability of secondary glaucoma.

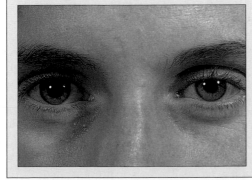

33 Left congenital Horner's syndrome – note the subtle iris heterochromia, ptosis and smaller pupil.

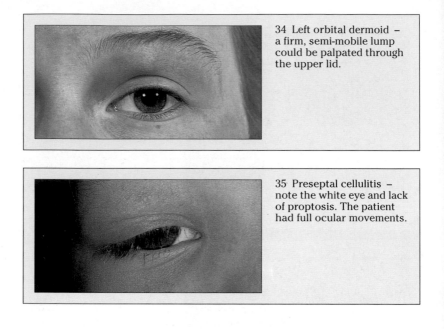

34 Left orbital dermoid – a firm, semi-mobile lump could be palpated through the upper lid.

35 Preseptal cellulitis – note the white eye and lack of proptosis. The patient had full ocular movements.

Orbital disorders (RARE)

Congenital structural abnormalities such as Crouzon's syndrome lead to characteristic dysmorphic features and often give rise to oculomotor abnormalities.

Orbital dermoids may present at any age as a smooth non-tender mass, usually in the superotemporal quadrant (**34**). They are often attached to periosteum and, as they may extend deep into the orbit, a computed tomography (CT) scan is useful.

Preseptal cellulitis arises from bacterial infection either spreading from a lid lesion such as a stye or infected chalazion, or following upper respiratory tract infection (**35**). The eye is white and the ocular movements are normal. *Orbital cellulitis* (an ophthalmic emergency) in children usually arises from one of the paranasal sinuses (see **146**). There is severe orbital congestion with lid oedema, conjunctival chemosis, restricted ocular movements, proptosis and sometimes reduced vision with an afferent pupil defect.

Orbital tumours often present with proptosis. This may arise relatively rapidly in the rare rhabdomyosarcoma, or more gradually in optic nerve gliomas, where an afferent pupil defect is likely to be present.

Does my child have a squint?

Strategy point – History
The best guide to a positive diagnosis in most cases is the mother. Ask about a family history of squint and/or amblyopia (lazy eye).

Strategy point – examination
Examine the corneal light reflexes and perform the cover and alternate cover tests. Beware the child with broad epicanthic folds giving a pseudosquint – rely on your tests.

Congenital convergent squint (RELATIVELY UNCOMMON)
The large angle of deviation and early onset make this diagnosis easy, and the differential diagnosis is effectively a bilateral VIth nerve palsy. The child with congenital convergent squint tends to have alternating fixation, using the right eye for looking left and vice versa. Test the ocular movements with one eye covered to establish if full movements can be achieved.

Convergent squints in older children (COMMON)
These are usually associated with hypermetropia and/or astigmatism. The eye with the greater *hypermetropia* and/or *astigmatism* is almost always the eye to become amblyopic (lazy) and therefore the one to converge (**36**). Convergence may only be demonstrated on accommodation in some children. Convergent squints are often associated with an overaction of the inferior oblique on horizontal movements, the adducting eye elevating, producing a vertical squint in that position of gaze.

Divergent squints in children (RELATIVELY UNCOMMON)
Most of these start by being intermittently divergent (careful history), and may appear initially straight on testing. The older child may admit to diplopia but younger children rapidly suppress the image from the diverg-

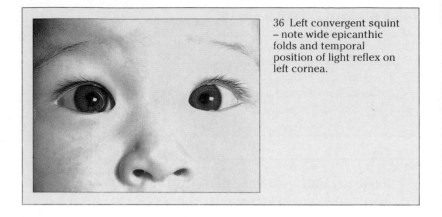

36 Left convergent squint – note wide epicanthic folds and temporal position of light reflex on left cornea.

ing eye. Dissociating the eyes with the cover test often induces the manifest squint which may or may not then be controllable by the child. The angle of squint assessed for distance, and particularly far distance, is almost always greater than that measured for near and significant optical errors and reduced acuities are unusual.

Strategy point – red reflexes
Once the squint has been diagnosed, it is essential to check the red reflexes as leukocoria (white pupil) requires urgent expert assessment.

Strategy point – cycloplegic refraction and fundoscopy
Accurate refraction is essential for the management of strabismus and amblyopia. An 'organic' cause for the squint must be excluded by fundoscopy.

The child that cannot see properly

Strategy point – History
Poor vision in one or both eyes may present as a result of vision screening at school (usually performed at age 5 years in school), or parental observation of abnormal visual behaviour. Occasionally the child (or teacher) notices reduced function compared with the child's peers. In general, children do not present with reduced vision in one eye unless formally tested as adaptation rapidly occurs, and the child functions normally with one good eye. Younger children also do not complain of bilateral reduced vision, particularly if the onset is relatively gradual.

Uniocular reduction in acuity
The most common cause is amblyopia in younger children (under 8 years of age) and late diagnosis of amblyopia and refractive errors in older children.

Strategy point – acuities and external appearance
How bad is the vision in the poor eye? Don't forget the pinhole in older children – a good result suggests a refractive error. Organic (non-amblyopic) causes of reduced acuity in one eye are rare and are usually detectable on clinical examination.

Strategy point – cover tests and red reflex
Look for a manifest squint with the cover test. The deviation may be very small if there is a microsquint with amblyopia.

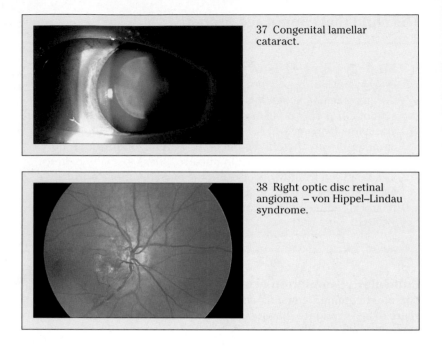

37 Congenital lamellar cataract.

38 Right optic disc retinal angioma – von Hippel–Lindau syndrome.

Exclude organic causes from front to back, checking cornea, iris, lens and vitreous. *Keratoconus* (see **75**) may rarely present in childhood, particularly in Down's syndrome, and is often very asymmetrical. *Congenital cataract* which has been missed in infancy may be uniocular (**37**). Vitreous opacities may be present as a result of chronic uveitis even in a white eye, or from vitreous haemorrhage secondary to congenital vascular abnormalities such as *von Hippel–Lindau syndrome* (**38**).

Strategy point
Pupils and (cycloplegic) refraction: If amblyopia is suspected, a refraction (under cycloplegia for younger children) is essential to determine any underlying optical error and the eye should look otherwise normal on clinical examination.

Strategy point – fundoscopy (all causes RARE)

Optic nerve glioma is usually uniocular, may cause a subtle proptosis (look for other stigmata of neurofibromatosis such as café-au-lait spots and *Lisch nodules* on the iris (**39**)) with an afferent pupil defect and optic atrophy. If the loss of vision is severe a divergent squint may occur.

Coloboma (congenital absence of tissue) of the optic nerve and/or retina (**40**) may be associated with other colobomata, particularly of the iris.

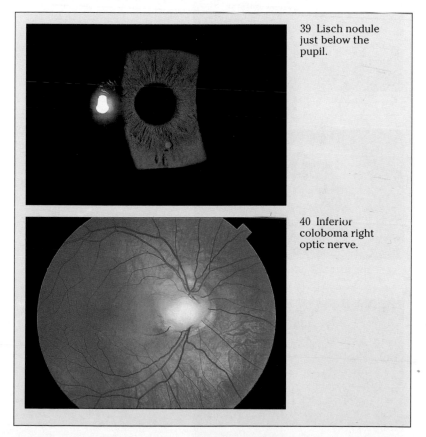

39 Lisch nodule just below the pupil.

40 Inferior coloboma right optic nerve.

Macular scarring may be as a result of *toxoplasmosis* (**41**) acquired in utero, toxocariasis or previous trauma. Massive retinal exudation from *Coats' disease* (**42**), much more common in males, may also present as a large retrolental mass simulating retinoblastoma.

Infiltration of the optic nerve from leukaemia is a rare acquired cause of poor vision (**43**).

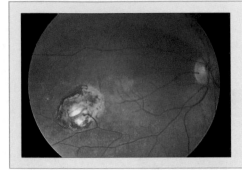

41 Extrafoveal toxoplasmosis scar – right eye. This patient was fortunate as this could easily have been on the fovea.

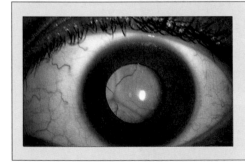

42 Exudative total retinal detachment seen through the pupil in an 11-year-old boy, fellow eye normal – Coats' disease.

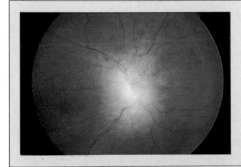

43 Leukaemic infiltration of right optic nerve. Acuity – light perception.

Binocular loss of vision (all causes RARE)

> **Strategy point**
> A similar strategy is followed as for uniocular visual loss.

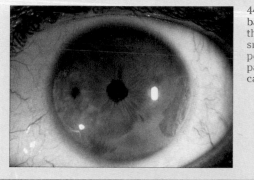

44 Still's disease – note band keratopathy sparing the central cornea and small irregular pupil from posterior synechiae. The patient also had significant cataract.

A pre- and perinatal history may suggest the diagnosis and must always be carefully taken. If bilateral poor vision is present from birth, and the level of corrected acuity is around 6/24 (20/80) or worse, nystagmus is likely to be present.

Look at the external eye – is it a normal size? Enlarged eyes may be as a result of congenital glaucoma whereas microphthalmos may result from chromosomal abnormalities, retinopathy of prematurity, congenital rubella or cytomegalovirus.

High refractive errors (myopia and hypermetropia) are a common cause of bilateral poor vision in children and must always be excluded by refraction following cycloplegia. Other causes are very rare in the developed world.

Anterior segment disorders such as corneal scarring from *Still's disease* (**44**) are detectable on direct illumination, and leukocoria from cataract and retinopathy of prematurity by the red reflex test. In certain parts of Africa and the East, vitamin A deficiency leads to corneal scarring and sometimes perforation, particularly when there is superadded measles infection (see Chapter 10).

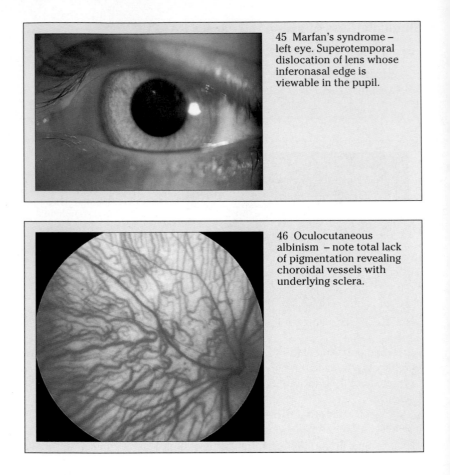

45 Marfan's syndrome – left eye. Superotemporal dislocation of lens whose inferonasal edge is viewable in the pupil.

46 Oculocutaneous albinism – note total lack of pigmentation revealing choroidal vessels with underlying sclera.

Bilateral congenital cataract of a relatively mild nature may reduce vision but not cause nystagmus. Opacities are usually limited to the central nuclear zone. *Lens dislocation*, as found most commonly in Marfan's syndrome (**45**), causes a progressive bilateral blurring, especially for distance. Both cataract and lens dislocation can be seen easily on examination of the red reflex, particularly when dilated.

Abnormalities of the retina associated with poor vision are multiple. In *albinism* (**46**), there is iris transillumination, foveal hypoplasia with nystagmus and the choroidal vessels are easily visible as little to no pigment can

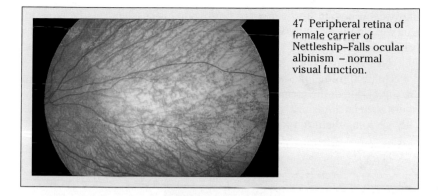

47 Peripheral retina of female carrier of Nettleship–Falls ocular albinism – normal visual function.

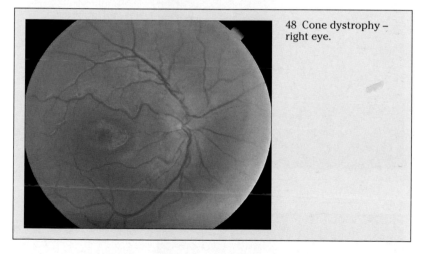

48 Cone dystrophy – right eye.

be seen in the fundus. The diagnosis is straightforward when the condition affects the whole body, but ocular forms exist. In *X-linked ocular albinism* (Nettleship–Falls), the typical signs are seen in the eyes of affected males, but with normal pigmentation elsewhere. Female carriers demonstrate mottled areas of hypopigmentation in the peripheral fundus (**47**).

Macular scarring may occur from *Stargardt's disease* (see **89**) (autosomal recessive, progressive visual loss, diffuse 'fish tail' yellowish-white flecks at the posterior pole and peripheral retina), and *cone dystrophy* (poor colour vision, 'bull's-eye' maculopathy) (**48**) or other rare retinal/pigment epithelial dystrophies. In *Best's disease* (autosomal recessive, relatively good acuity in childhood with preserved colour vision, poor EOG) (**49**), there is a characteristic 'egg yolk' appearance at the macula which 'scrambles' with time (**50**). Vision in the former stage is remarkably preserved.

Peripheral retinal pigmentation of a 'bone spicule' nature is usually as a result of one of the forms of *retinitis pigmentosa (RP)* (**51**). RP is usually inherited in an autosomal recessive manner when it presents in childhood, with a 'clumsy' child, particularly in dim lighting. A more severe form

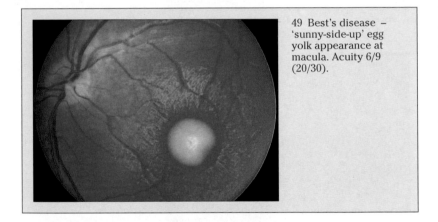

49 Best's disease –
'sunny-side-up' egg
yolk appearance at
macula. Acuity 6/9
(20/30).

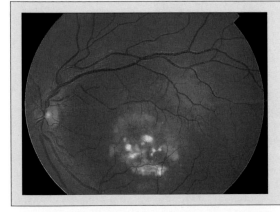

50 Best's disease –
'scrambled' macula
appearance – vision
6/36 (20/120).

(Leber's amaurosis) presents in infancy with a blind child with nystagmus, externally normal eyes and little abnormal to see on fundoscopy. The main differential diagnosis of Leber's amaurosis is 'delayed visual maturation' in which visual function improves with time and the flash electroretinogram is grossly normal.

Optic disc abnormalities associated with bilateral poor vision include optic nerve hypoplasia (**52**), familial optic atrophy, optic disc swelling from inflammation, or severe papilloedema.

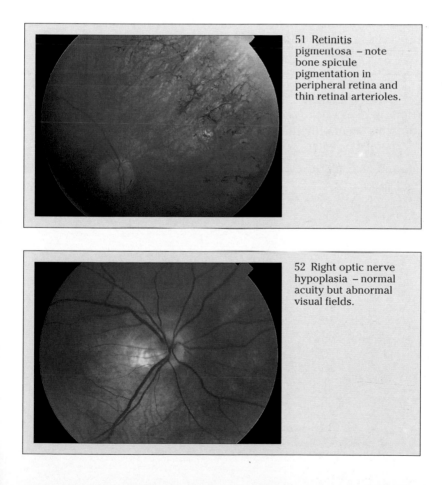

51 Retinitis pigmentosa – note bone spicule pigmentation in peripheral retina and thin retinal arterioles.

52 Right optic nerve hypoplasia – normal acuity but abnormal visual fields.

Hysterical visual loss in children (RARE)

This may present in a number of ways. Following a relatively minor head injury a young child may deny vision in one or both eyes for a period of time. More commonly there appears to be no precipitating cause, the child is older, around 10–14 years of age, and usually female. If suspected, a number of tests may be used to confirm the diagnosis, such as rotating a mirror in front of the child if 'total blindness' is claimed (the child's eyes move as the mirror rotates), and using 'correcting' lenses, the optics of which when combined are neutral, to 'improve the vision'. Visual field testing often produces a restriction that worsens as the test proceeds (a spiral field).

Strategy point

It is advisable to seek a paediatric opinion when visual problems occur other than as a result of refractive errors and non-paralytic squint.

CHAPTER 4
CHRONIC LOSS OF VISION

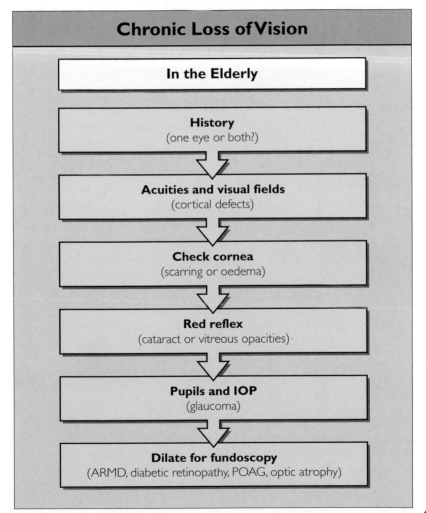

Chronic Loss of Vision

In the Elderly

History
(one eye or both?)

Acuities and visual fields
(cortical defects)

Check cornea
(scarring or oedema)

Red reflex
(cataract or vitreous opacities)

Pupils and IOP
(glaucoma)

Dilate for fundoscopy
(ARMD, diabetic retinopathy, POAG, optic atrophy)

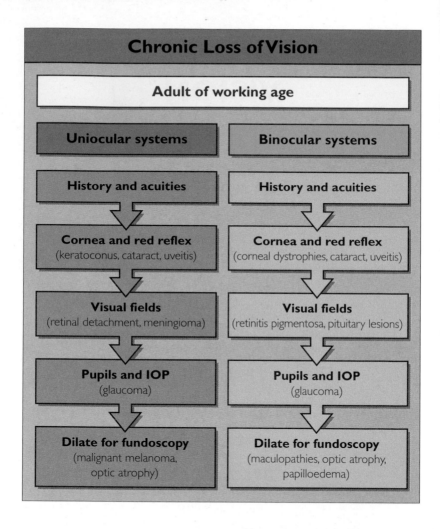

Chronic Loss of Vision

Adult of working age

Uniocular systems	Binocular systems
History and acuities	**History and acuities**
Cornea and red reflex (keratoconus, cataract, uveitis)	**Cornea and red reflex** (corneal dystrophies, cataract, uveitis)
Visual fields (retinal detachment, meningioma)	**Visual fields** (retinitis pigmentosa, pituitary lesions)
Pupils and IOP (glaucoma)	**Pupils and IOP** (glaucoma)
Dilate for fundoscopy (malignant melanoma, optic atrophy)	**Dilate for fundoscopy** (maculopathies, optic atrophy, papilloedema)

Definition of chronic loss of vision

Chronic loss of vision indicates symptoms which have come on gradually over the course of weeks or months rather than minutes, hours or a few days.

Strategy point – the History
Chronic loss of vision is almost always painless. The first aspect to explore is whether the symptoms are uniocular or binocular (and if the latter, any asymmetry?), and their duration. Is the visual defect predominantly central (e.g. from macular degeneration), or global (e.g. cataract). Always take a history of previous ocular disease, present medications, ocular and systemic, and ask especially about amblyopia, diabetes and hypertension. A positive family history of glaucoma prompts careful exclusion of this disorder.

The elderly patient with chronic loss of vision

Chronic loss of vision in the elderly is often binocular but asymmetrical, the patient only complaining of the worse eye unless vision is also significantly reduced in the better eye.

Strategy point
Measure the vision for near and distance in each eye (don't forget the pinhole), then quickly check the visual fields by confrontation for gross defects. (The detection of post-chiasmal disease at this stage in the examination changes the course of the consultation, promoting further questions relevant to the findings.)

Homonomous hemianopia (UNUSUAL)
A cerebrovascular accident causing ocular symptoms usually gives a homonomous hemianopia (HH) that is easily detectable by confrontation. A good history leads the doctor to the diagnosis, but elderly patients often confuse a loss of vision on one side (HH) with loss of vision in the eye on that side. Remember too, in a total right HH that is dense, distance acuity is good but reading acuity is very poor (one cannot scan into a macular splitting scotoma). Macular sparing in a complete hemianopia indicates an occipital cortex lesion. In cortical blindness from bilateral infarcts, the eyes (including optic discs) are normal, as are the pupil reflexes.

Strategy point

It is wise to aim to exclude each of the 'big three' – cataract, macular degeneration and chronic simple glaucoma (CSG) (or in a diabetic, the big four with retinopathy) in every elderly patient. Remember, they often coexist and one must be careful not to attribute all the symptoms to the first sign detected.

Strategy point

Check the cornea with the pen torch for opacities or oedema which would affect the red reflex (e.g. band keratopathy or scarring). (Symptomatic *Fuch's endothelial dystrophy* in its early stages appears as epithelial bedewing on slit lamp examination. Later, stromal oedema is shown well by scleral scatter; **53**.)

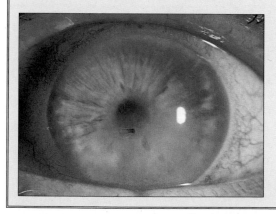

53 Fuch's endothelial dystrophy – advanced stage. Some epithelial breakdown occurring inferiorly.

Corneal scarring as a cause of reduced vision (RARE)

If bilateral and diffuse, congenital syphilis is considered (look for the saddle nose and Hutchinson's teeth). Unilateral cases may be secondary to previous *herpes simplex* (**54**), herpes zoster ophthalmicus, or ocular trauma.

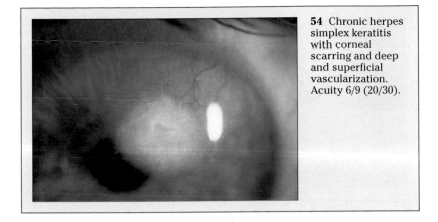

54 Chronic herpes simplex keratitis with corneal scarring and deep and superficial vascularization. Acuity 6/9 (20/30).

Strategy point

To detect cataract, examine the red reflex and next test the pupils (established CSG usually gives a RAPD on the worse side).

Cataract (COMMON)

The position and nature of the opacity determines the symptoms and vision under differing circumstances. Posterior capsule thickening following cataract surgery is considered where appropriate.

Nuclear sclerosis

This produces an artificial refractive myopia, progressively blurring distance vision but preserving near vision until dense. The opacity is seen as a globular dimness centrally on red reflex when pupil dilated or as a progressive central yellowing with oblique illumination (**55**).

Cortical

This reduces distance vision mainly in the early stages with dazzling in bright lights or when driving at night. Seen as opacities like the spokes of a wheel in one or more quadrants on red reflex (**56**). The opacities appear white on slit lamp examination, usually in the peripheral cortex.

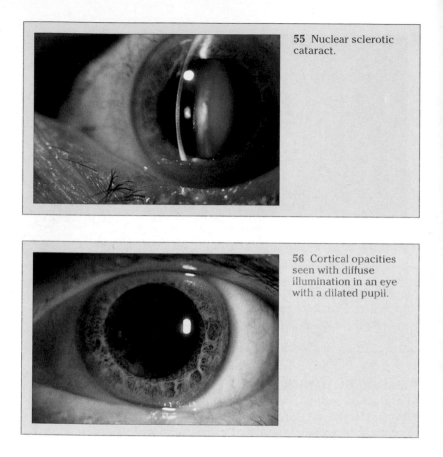

55 Nuclear sclerotic cataract.

56 Cortical opacities seen with diffuse illumination in an eye with a dilated pupil.

Posterior subcapsular

The worst vision is when the pupil is small, i.e. in bright lighting and when reading. Undilated, the red reflex may be abolished when viewing axially, but after dilation the central position of the opacity is clear. The granular opacity just under the posterior capsule is best appreciated by retroillumination (direct the slit beam perpendicular to the cornea and view against the red reflex) (**57**).

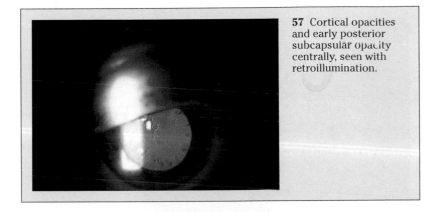

57 Cortical opacities and early posterior subcapsular opacity centrally, seen with retroillumination.

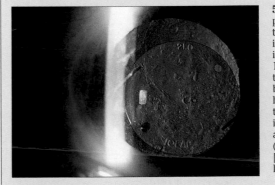

58 Significant posterior capsule thickening following intraocular lens implantation. This 1980s style implant has two polypropylene blue loops, two dialling holes and the power of the lens clearly imprinted on it. Visual acuity 6/36 (20/120) (improved to 6/6 [20/20] following Yag laser capsulotomy).

Posterior capsule thickening

This complication occurs in about 20% of eyes within five years of cataract surgery (**58**). It may reduce vision out of proportion to the physical signs because of its position. Some elderly patients may have forgotten that they have had cataract surgery to the eye in the past, and with modern surgical techniques, it can be difficult to identify if surgery has taken place. The opacities are best seen following dilation and are most easily visualized by examining the red reflex with a direct ophthalmoscope, focusing on the capsule, or by retroillumination on the slit lamp.

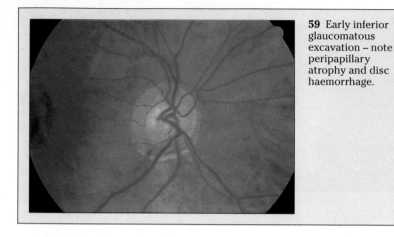

59 Early inferior glaucomatous excavation – note peripapillary atrophy and disc haemorrhage.

Strategy point
Test the intraocular pressure (IOP). Then dilate the pupil and examine the disc and macula.

Glaucomatous optic atrophy (COMMON)
In the Western world progressive *open angle glaucoma* (POAG) now only rarely presents as reduced reading vision, most cases being detected at an earlier stage by screening. However, it often coexists with cataract or macular degeneration.

The cardinal sign is disc excavation – a progressive enlargement of the optic cup, with consequent thinning of the neuroretinal rim (**59**).

Unless detected by screening, patients may not present until advanced disease is present in at least one eye as chronic glaucoma rarely affects central vision until almost all of the peripheral field has been extinguished. In advanced disease, the neuroretinal rim is severely thinned and pale and the cup occupies most of the disc area. The position of the edge of the cup is most easily delineated by an angulation of the blood vessels as they pass over the edge of the rim. It is not unusual for a disc in this stage to be errantly considered 'flat' when viewed with a direct

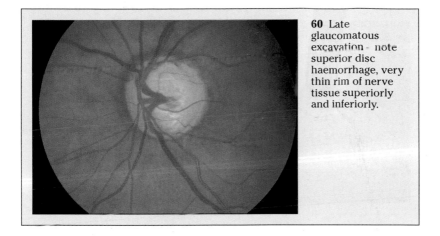

60 Late glaucomatous excavation - note superior disc haemorrhage, very thin rim of nerve tissue superiorly and inferiorly.

ophthalmoscope. The size and shape of the cup is best determined by a contact lens or 90/78/60 dioptre lens examination using a thin, vertically orientated slit beam passed slowly across the disc.

In less advanced disease, the rim is still pink and the diagnosis is best made by observing the shape of the cup. In glaucoma, a previously round or horizontally oval cup becomes vertically oval, thinning particularly at the inferotemporal rim. A disc haemorrhage (**60**) may aid the diagnosis, as may the presence of peripapillary atrophy where the sclera is visible around the disc (this must not be confused with a scleral crescent found in myopia).

Age-related macular degeneration (ARMD) (COMMON)

The acute 'disciform' variety of this disorder is discussed elsewhere. In the *chronic dry* variety, there is a slow bilateral reduction in central vision, initially having its main effect on reading, particularly in dim light. The patient may notice gaps in words with one eye closed and later with both eyes open. Often the request is for 'stronger reading glasses'.

On examination of the fundus a variety of signs may be seen:

- Drusen – these are distinct round/oval yellowish bodies scattered over the macula. Occasionally they are misdiagnosed as hard exudates. Exudates are whiter, and less uniformly distributed, usually being associated with microvascular abnormalities. In some patients the drusen

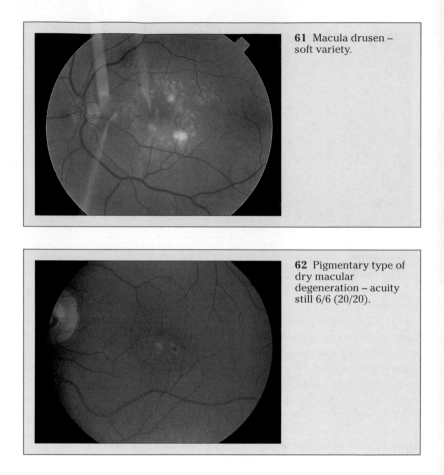

61 Macula drusen – soft variety.

62 Pigmentary type of dry macular degeneration – acuity still 6/6 (20/20).

appear larger and soft edged (**61**), as though coalescence has taken place – these eyes are at increased risk of acute disciform formation.

- Hyper/hypopigmentation (**62**) – seen in varying degrees over the macula. Often seen with drusen.
- Macular pucker – less common than the above and more difficult to see. Patients have a chronic distortion of central vision from a gliotic glistening membrane over the macula. Perifoveal capillaries may appear more tortuous than normal and there is a loss of the normal foveal reflex (**63**). A slit beam accentuates the puckering of the internal

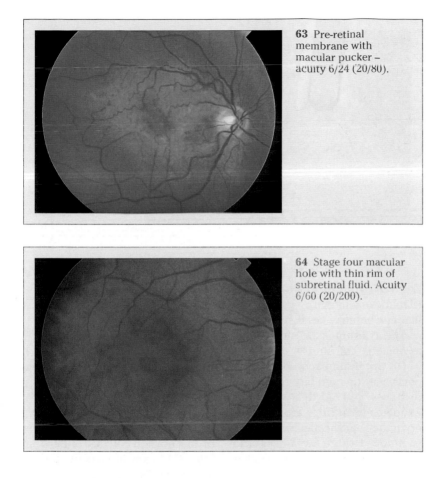

63 Pre-retinal membrane with macular pucker – acuity 6/24 (20/80).

64 Stage four macular hole with thin rim of subretinal fluid. Acuity 6/60 (20/200).

limiting membrane.
- Macular hole – again rarer and more difficult to see – usually unilateral but careful examination of the fellow eye is essential to exclude early changes which may be reversible by surgery. A vision of 6/24 (20/80)or worse is found in established cases with a round red punched-out appearance to the centre of the fovea, with yellow pigment spots some-times visible at the base. A degree of subretinal fluid accumulation may be observable with the slit beam (**64**), and cystoid changes surrounding the circular 'hole' should make one suspect a lamellar or pseudohole.

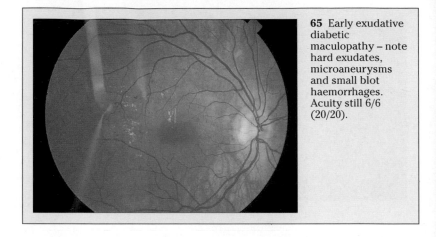

65 Early exudative diabetic maculopathy – note hard exudates, microaneurysms and small blot haemorrhages. Acuity still 6/6 (20/20).

Diabetic maculopathy (COMMON)

Diabetic maculopathy usually is suspected if the patient is known to be diabetic but may be the presenting feature in diabetes.

The symptoms are similar to those of ARMD, but often with greater asymmetry and shorter duration.

On ophthalmoscopy the common findings are exudates, microaneurysms, dot and blot haemorrhages (**65**), and sometimes flame haemorrhages and cotton wool spots around the posterior pole (**66**). Exudates form rings around microvascular abnormalities, often lining up in the superficial nerve fibre layer around the fovea. When the vision is reduced there usually is a loss of the normal foveal reflex from oedema. Oedema is best visualized with a slit beam and a contact lens, although it can often be appreciated with the 78 dioptre and similar lenses (**67**).

Strategy point

Check the colour vision and perform careful confrontation fields if optic atrophy is suspected.

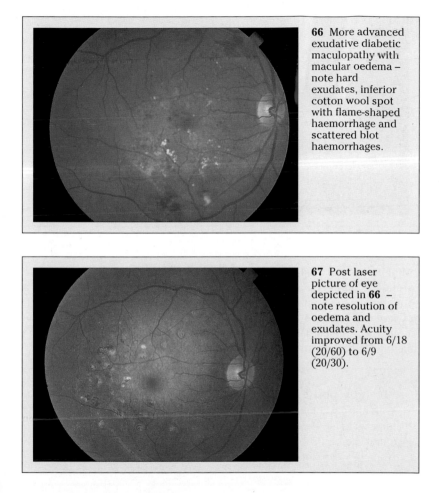

66 More advanced exudative diabetic maculopathy with macular oedema – note hard exudates, inferior cotton wool spot with flame-shaped haemorrhage and scattered blot haemorrhages.

67 Post laser picture of eye depicted in **66** – note resolution of oedema and exudates. Acuity improved from 6/18 (20/60) to 6/9 (20/30).

Flat optic atrophy (RARE)

A bilateral symmetrical reduction in acuity, recording anywhere between 6/9 (20/30) to 6/60 (20/200) in both eyes (**68**), with optic atrophy and poor colour vision would prompt questions on diet, smoking and alcohol ingestion for a diagnosis of nutritional amblyopia, or vitamin B_{12} deficiency (secondary to gastrectomy or pernicious anaemia). Heavy-metal poisoning and drug toxicity are also considered.

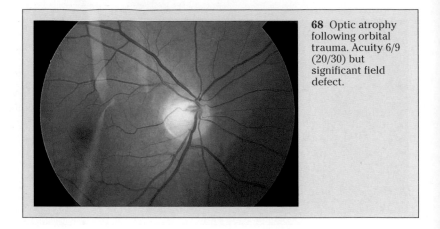

68 Optic atrophy following orbital trauma. Acuity 6/9 (20/30) but significant field defect.

If a peripheral field defect is detected in one eye, check the other eye carefully; compressive lesions close to the chiasm anteriorly, such as a sphenoidal wing meningioma, may cause a profound defect in the ipsilateral eye (with flat optic atrophy) and a small peripheral scotoma in the fellow eye. An unexplained field defect merits a CT or magnetic resonance imaging (MRI) scan to exclude a compressive lesion.

Strategy point

With normal colour vision but optic atrophy, suspect glaucoma and look again for excavation. This is particularly likely in a small disc which has a bowed back appearance on three-dimensional slit beam examination.

Combined pathology (COMMON)

The big three (cataract, macular degeneration and progressive open angle glaucoma) often coexist in an elderly patient. It is particularly important not to attribute visual loss which is out of proportion to the physical signs, to early cataract without a full examination. It is surprising how well one can visualize the fundus with a direct ophthalmoscope in a patient with early cataract if good pupillary dilation is achieved.

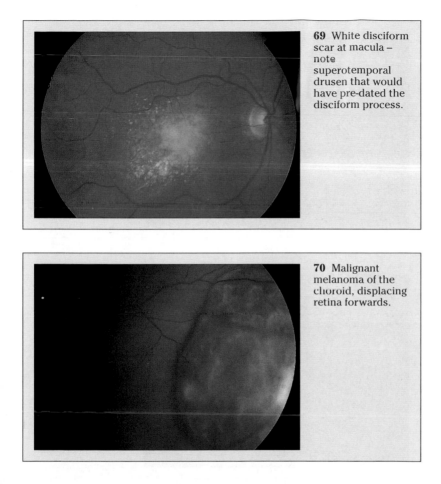

69 White disciform scar at macula – note superotemporal drusen that would have pre-dated the disciform process.

70 Malignant melanoma of the choroid, displacing retina forwards.

Other fundal lesions (disciform COMMON; others RARE)

Fundal examination often reveals pathology that requires diagnosis. The lesion(s) may be asymptomatic or be reducing visual function. Raised lesions often cause concern. A large macular scar from an *old disciform* (see Chapter 5) may be raised and appear like a white 'tumour' (**69**). *Malignant melanomas* of the choroid (**70**) may present with a variety of appearances from a relatively flat grey lesion, superficially similar to a

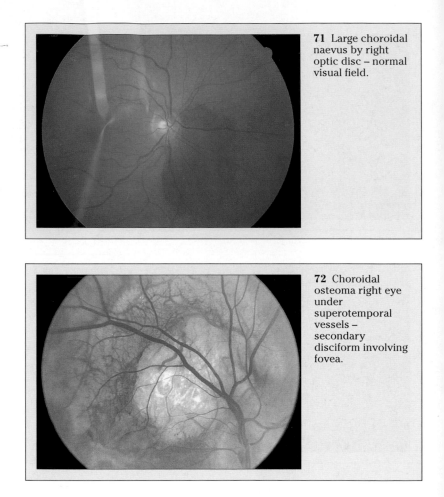

71 Large choroidal naevus by right optic disc – normal visual field.

72 Choroidal osteoma right eye under superotemporal vessels – secondary disciform involving fovea.

naevus (**71**), to a large multiloculated lesion with secondary retinal detachment. *Choroidal secondaries* are usually multiple, pale in colour and bilateral. By contrast, the very rare *choroidal osteoma* (**72, 73**) is single, usually outside the macula, and has a characteristic high-reflectance echo on ultrasound due to calcification within the lesion. A very dark grey, flat lesion, usually in the retinal periphery and

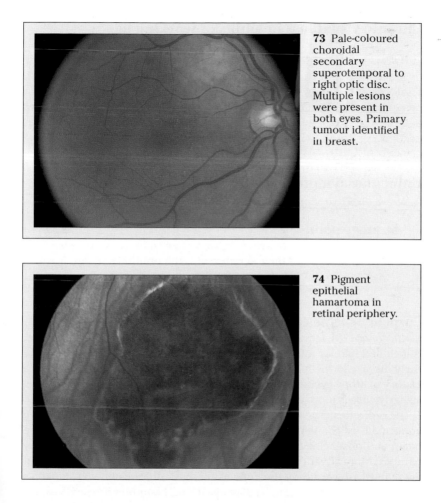

73 Pale-coloured choroidal secondary superotemporal to right optic disc. Multiple lesions were present in both eyes. Primary tumour identified in breast.

74 Pigment epithelial hamartoma in retinal periphery.

surrounded by a 'halo' of white sclera characterizes the *retinal pigment epithelial hamartoma* (**74**).

Nothing abnormal?

Suspect a poor performance with the pinhole and test again. Refer to a specialist for a second opinion if in doubt.

Chronic visual loss in adults of working age

Early-onset, age-related changes (COMMON) (e.g. cataract and macular degeneration and diabetic retinopathy) must be considered IN ALL CASES as age increases, but another collection of pathologies must also be kept in mind, and these are discussed in this section. In the younger person, the history is more likely to be accurate and must be taken particularly carefully.

Uniocular symptoms

Strategy point
Exclude media opacities first with a pen torch for the cornea and then examination of the red reflex with the ophthalmoscope.

Corneal opacities (RARE)
Keratoconus (**75**), a dystrophic ectasia with thinning of the central cornea, is included here as it frequently presents with uniocular blurring despite early disease in the fellow eye. Presenting in the late teens to twenties, a history of atopy is common. Traditionally diagnosed with a Placido's disc, an early case is more easily diagnosed by the typical globular shape seen in the red reflex. The corneal position of this defect in the reflex can be confirmed by changing the angle of incidence of the ophthalmoscope beam and observing the change in relative position of the 'globule' by parallax. More advanced cases can be diagnosed by observing the indent made in the lower lid by the cone as the patient looks down (Munson's sign). Very subtle cases can be diagnosed with computer assisted corneal topography.

Cataract (COMMON)
Uniocular cataract prompts questions on previous trauma and an examination to find the cause.

In *Fuch's heterochromic cyclitis* (**76**) the iris on the affected side is of lighter colour and the cataract is posterior subcapsular before progressing

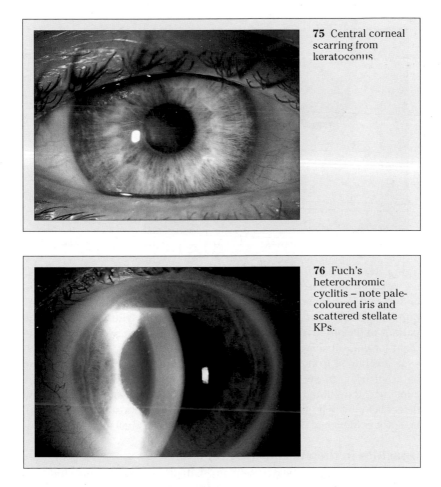

75 Central corneal scarring from keratoconus

76 Fuch's heterochromic cyclitis – note pale-coloured iris and scattered stellate KPs.

to a dense white lens (stellate keratic precipitates are evenly distributed on the endothelium, cells may be present in the anterior chamber and anterior vitreous, and dilated iris vessels may be seen. Posterior synechiae are never found).

Remember – a posterior subcapsular cataract may be the result of chronic local steroid instillation.

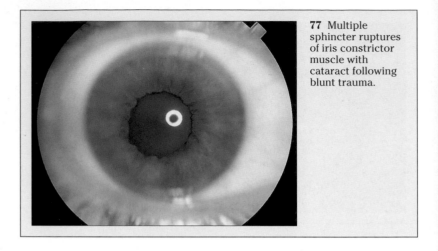

77 Multiple sphincter ruptures of iris constrictor muscle with cataract following blunt trauma.

In cataract related to *blunt trauma*, there may be signs of iris damage, e.g. a pupil which is larger or smaller than its fellow, an efferent pupil defect, and perhaps iridodialysis. Look for sphincter ruptures around the pupil margin (**77**) and for iridodynesis and lenticulodynesis by asking the patient to flick their eyes from side to side, pausing between each movement for your observation.

In a retained iron-containing *intraocular foreign body* (IOFB; **78**), the cataract is often stellate, with ferrous deposits on the anterior lens capsule. A combined afferent (from retinal toxicity) and efferent pupil defect is found in a rusty brown iris (from iron salt deposition – siderosis). Look for evidence of previous IOFB entry such as a small defect in the iris.

Opacities in the vitreous (RARE)

A chronic uniocular uveitis usually presents as chronic floaters (but may cause loss of vision from band keratopathy, secondary cataract, secondary glaucoma, cystoid macular oedema or chronic hypotony with choroidal folds). The eye may well be white and therefore other signs of uveitis must be sought, e.g. posterior synechiae and keratic precipitates. Occasionally, *asteroid hyalosis* (**79**) causes visual symptoms (posterior vitrectomy has been performed for this condition). Fundal examination is very difficult because of the deposits suspended in the vitreous. It is associated with diabetes. In scintesis scintillans similar deposits gravitate inferiorly following ocular movements.

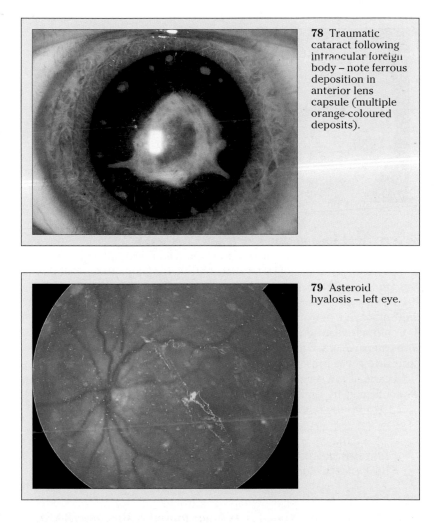

78 Traumatic cataract following intraocular foreign body – note ferrous deposition in anterior lens capsule (multiple orange-coloured deposits).

79 Asteroid hyalosis – left eye.

Strategy point
Now perform a confrontation field.

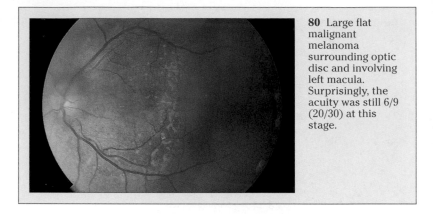

80 Large flat malignant melanoma surrounding optic disc and involving left macula. Surprisingly, the acuity was still 6/9 (20/30) at this stage.

Severe field loss in one eye (FAIRLY RARE)

A total loss of vision in an area of the field which extends to the periphery, particularly if in a superior distribution, indicates the possibility of *long-standing retinal detachment* (see **114**). These are usually inferiorly sited (superior detachments tend to progress rapidly) and may only present when macular function has been compromised.

Compressive lesions such as sphenoidal wing meningioma may present with extensive uniocular field loss despite only minimal acuity reduction – optic atrophy is present.

Occasionally, a very asymmetrical severe glaucoma presents thus and can be confirmed by optic disc assessment. Suspect a traumatic aetiology, pseudoexfoliation or iridocorneoendothelial dystrophy.

> **Strategy point**
> Check the IOP and pupil responses, and then dilate.

Chronic uniocular visual loss from macular disease (RARE)

A relatively flat *malignant melanoma* (**80**) involving the macula may cause a slow deterioration of vision, as can *radiation retinopathy* following treatment for malignant disease (see **240**). Macular oedema may also result from *perifoveal capillary telangectasia* of unknown origin (**81**). Pigment epitheliopathies may present with uniocular symptoms, but the signs are usually bilateral.

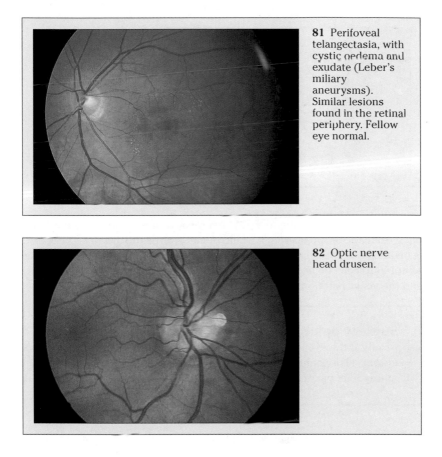

81 Perifoveal telangectasia, with cystic oedema and exudate (Leber's miliary aneurysms). Similar lesions found in the retinal periphery. Fellow eye normal.

82 Optic nerve head drusen.

Optic nerve-related uniocular visual loss (RARE)

Uniocular *optic atrophy* with chronic loss of vision requires careful investigation as the cause must be considered to be a space-occupying lesion such as an anterior cerebral artery aneurysm or meningioma until proven otherwise. Shunt vessels on the disc make the diagnosis of optic nerve sheath meningioma likely, whereas an altitudinal field defect and a small disc with a knobbly, irregular outline suggests *optic nerve head drusen* (**82**). (This is invariably binocular, although it often presents with uniocular symptoms.) Drusen may autofluoresce (look down the fluorescein camera) but are best confirmed by ultrasonography.

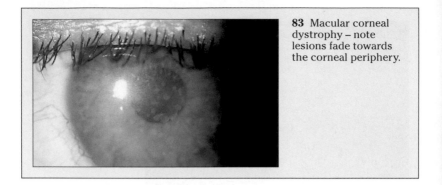

83 Macular corneal dystrophy – note lesions fade towards the corneal periphery.

Very occasionally, dysthyroid optic neuropathy may be uniocular and without a dramatic proptosis which would point towards the diagnosis. The disc is oedematous with engorged veins. Other signs of dysthyroid disease, such as conjunctival chemosis and restrictive ophthalmopathy, must be sought, and the visual function of the fellow eye must be scrutinized carefully.

Strategy point
Finally, if the eye looks unequivocally normal and so are the field, colour vision and pupils, suspect a long-standing childhood amblyopia, particularly if the patient has anisometropia.

Binocular symptoms

Strategy point
Again, first exclude media opacities.

Corneal disease (RARE)
Symmetrical corneal opacities occur in a number of *corneal stromal dystrophies* (**83**) which disturb vision to varying degrees. The position and morphology of the deposits define the diagnosis with macular (autosomal

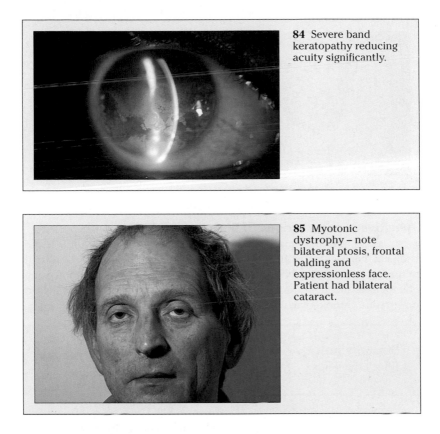

84 Severe band keratopathy reducing acuity significantly.

85 Myotonic dystrophy – note bilateral ptosis, frontal balding and expressionless face. Patient had bilateral cataract.

dominant) having the greatest effect on vision. *Band keratopathy* (**84**) in the absence of other ocular disease would suggest hypercalcaemia or Still's disease.

Cataract (COMMON)

In the younger age group bilateral cataract suggests diabetes or an inherited tendency to 'presenile cataract' if the morphology is indistinguishable from those seen in the elderly. Chronic systemic (or inhaled) steroids induce posterior subcapsular opacities. Other causes include *myotonic dystrophy* (distinguished by the male pattern baldness, bilateral ptosis and 'blank' expression), and hypoparathyroidism (**85**).

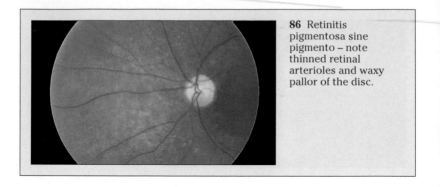

86 Retinitis pigmentosa sine pigmento – note thinned retinal arterioles and waxy pallor of the disc.

Opacities in the vitreous of both eyes (RARE)

Pars planitis, an inflammation of the peripheral retina and ciliary body, results in 'hazy vision with floaters' in young adults. (Sometimes it is found on routine examination.) Dilated examination of the peripheral retina using indentation with an indirect ophthalmoscope reveals 'snowball' opacities in the vitreous. Cystoid macula oedema may be the main cause of loss of acuity.

Strategy point
Check the fields.

Binocular field defects causing chronic visual loss (RARE)

In chronic chiasmal disease, when bitemporal field loss is advanced, central acuity may be affected. Patients may not notice even a pronounced field defect due to preservation of both nasal fields and, unless the field is tested, the diagnosis may be delayed. With a pituitary tumour (the classical lesion from below) the bitemporal hemianopia is most dense superiorly, whereas with a craniopharyngioma (with pressure from above) the defect is predominantly inferiorly sited. Optic atrophy is present in severe cases but not in all.

If the fields are uniformly constricted, suspect *retinitis pigmentosa* (**86**). Symptoms of night blindness usually precede complaints of poor side and later central vision. A posterior subcapsular cataract may be found, but the major signs are on fundoscopy – optic atrophy, thinned major blood vessels and 'bone spicule' pigmentation of the peripheral retina.

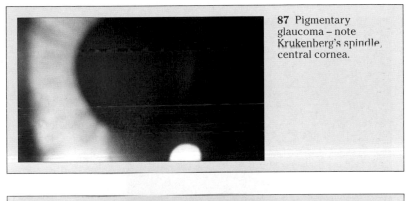

87 Pigmentary glaucoma – note Krukenberg's spindle, central cornea.

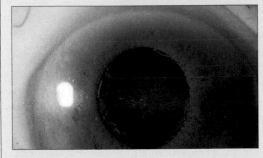

88 Pseudoexfoliation of the lens seen following dilation of the pupil – note dandruff-like deposits on the anterior lens capsule just within the pupil margin.

Strategy point

Now check the IOP and pupils and dilate.

Glaucoma in the under-65s (RARE, but COMMONER in some races)

Visual loss from *chronic simple glaucoma* in a younger patient is more common in black patients.

In whites, severe glaucoma at a relatively early age is often 'secondary'. The most common of these is *pigmentary glaucoma* (**87**) and *pseudoexfoliation of the lens* (**88**). The former is found more commonly in young (aged 20–40 years) male myopes, whereas the latter is often found in those from

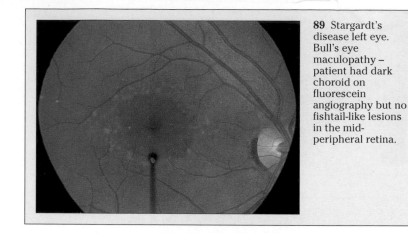

89 Stargardt's disease left eye. Bull's eye maculopathy – patient had dark choroid on fluorescein angiography but no fishtail-like lesions in the mid-peripheral retina.

Scandinavian origin. Since these diseases may be advanced before the age where routine screening commences, patients may present with severe field defects and sometimes acuity loss. One of the cardinal signs of pigment dispersion is Krukenberg's spindle, a vertical line of pigment deposits centrally placed on the endothelium. The iris shows a number of more subtle signs: peripheral slit transillumination defects, deposits of free pigment on its surface, and a typical reverse bombe effect in the periphery – best appreciated at gonioscopy.

Maculopathies (COMMON)

Bilateral macular disease in the younger adult gives similar symptoms and signs to those that occur in the older patient, with *diabetic maculopathy* exceeding age-related changes in frequency. There are some rarer but well-recognized disorders. *Best's disease* (see **49, 50**) and *Stargardt's disease* (**89**) may present in adult life. *Central choroidal sclerosis* (**90**), a dominant or recessive disorder often presenting in the fourth and fifth decade of life, appears as a punched-out loss of central pigment epithelium and chorio-capillaris, revealing the larger choroidal vessels and white sclera.

Other pigmentary maculopathies may occur as a result of chronic drug ingestion, a careful history being mandatory in such cases. Examples of agents with potential toxic effects are chloroquine, thioridizine and tamoxifen.

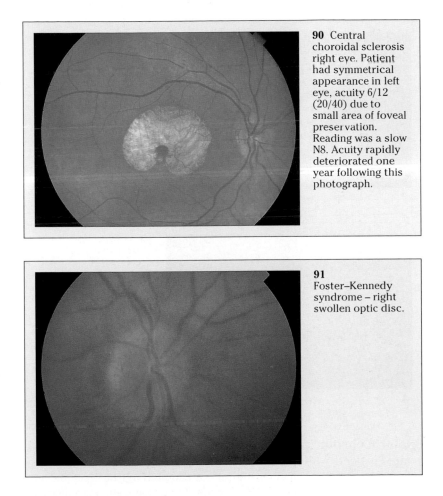

90 Central choroidal sclerosis right eye. Patient had symmetrical appearance in left eye, acuity 6/12 (20/40) due to small area of foveal preservation. Reading was a slow N8. Acuity rapidly deteriorated one year following this photograph.

91 Foster–Kennedy syndrome – right swollen optic disc.

Bilateral optic atrophy (RARE)

Bilateral flat optic atrophy requires exclusion of toxic and compressive causes as in the elderly.

The *Foster–Kennedy syndrome* is worthy of mention here. Optic atrophy in one eye is associated with papilloedema in the fellow eye and usually indicates a large meningioma of the sphenoid (**91, 92**). (A grossly atrophic nerve cannot become swollen from raised intracranial pressure.)

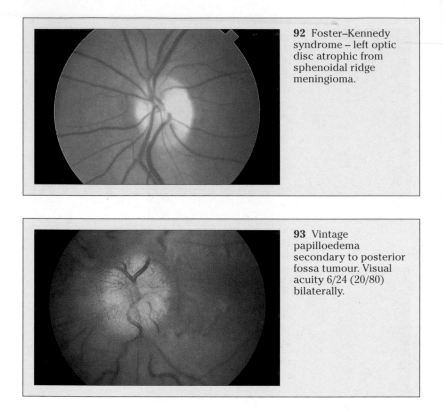

92 Foster–Kennedy syndrome – left optic disc atrophic from sphenoidal ridge meningioma.

93 Vintage papilloedema secondary to posterior fossa tumour. Visual acuity 6/24 (20/80) bilaterally.

Bilateral chronic papilloedema (RARE)

In most patients with papilloedema (disc swelling secondary to raised intracranial pressure), ocular symptoms are limited to transient obscurations of vision (see Chapter 5). However, when chronic and extreme as in *'vintage papilloedema'* (**93**), secondary ischaemic changes at the optic nerve head reduce acuity.

Benign intracranial hypertension (found typically in overweight young females with long-standing headache) may present with chronic loss of vision despite moderate papilloedema. An inter-eye red desaturation is often present and in addition to enlarged blind spots, other field defects are similar to those found in chronic glaucoma. The CT scan should be normal for this diagnosis to be entertained.

CHAPTER 5

ACUTE PAINLESS VISUAL DISTURBANCE

Acute visual loss			
Uniocular		**Binocular**	
Central	*Peripheral*	*Central*	*Peripheral*
Retinal ARMD Vein and arterial occlusion CSR	**Retinal** Detachment Retinal migraine CMV retinitis	**Retinal** CMV retinitis AMPPE Hypertension	**Retinal** Detachment
Optic nerve Optic neuritis Ischaemic ON	**Optic nerve** Ischaemic ON	**Optic nerve** Infiltrative Vintage papilloedema	**Optic nerve** Drusen
Media opacity Vitreous haemorrhage Choroiditis		**Cortical** Infarction Hysteria	**Cortical** Homonomous Bitemporal
Adie's syndrome			

Acute visual disturbances and diplopia				
Uniocular			**Binocular**	
Amaurosis	*Intrusions*	*Diplopia*	*Disturbances*	*Diplopia*
Emboli Arteritis	Floaters Entoptic	Cataract Chalazion	Migraine Raised ICP	Horizontal Vertical Mixed

Definition of acute visual loss and disturbance

This chapter deals with disorders of visual function which are painless and which have a well-defined onset.

Strategy point – The History

Taking the time to take an accurate history is of great importance in the patient who presents with acute visual disturbance. Full details of all symptoms that are volunteered are carefully explored. Most patients are elderly and often it is necessary to ask supplementary questions to ensure that the correct examination strategy is embarked upon from the outset.

The answers to the following questions are always sought:

1. Is it one eye or both?
2. Are the symptoms intermittent or constant?
3. If constant, are they improving, worsening or static?
4. Is all of the vision effected?

Details of past ocular history, past medical history and drug ingestion, including alcohol and smoking, are essential.

Strategy point

Check the acuities and test the fields. This leads to eight basic scenarios:

Uniocular   *Binocular*

predominantly central loss

predominantly peripheral field loss

normal acuities and fields

diplopia

> **Strategy point**
> Check the pupils then dilate, except when diplopia is the main symptom. Most of the diagnoses to be entertained are posterior segment or neuro-ophthalmological. Finding an afferent pupil defect indicates severe retinal dysfunction or optic nerve disease.

Uniocular predominantly central visual loss: normal pupils

Macular and paramacular disease (COMMON)

Disease limited to the macula and/or one sector of the retina only rarely affects the pupils (cf. optic nerve disease).

An important symptom in macular disease is central distortion, with straight lines appearing bent, wavy or having gaps in them. Visual acuity may vary from 6/6 (20/20) to Count Fingers (CF) in macular disease depending on the severity of disruption to retinal photoreceptors. Macular assessment is best performed with the slit lamp and one of the high-powered condensing lenses which give a binocular view of the fundus, preferably a contact lens, which facilitates angular slit beam illumination. However, careful examination with the direct ophthalmoscope often allows the diagnosis to be made.

In the older adult, from age 60 onwards, central distortion usually indicates acute *age-related macular degeneration* of the 'disciform' variety or its variant, pigment epithelial detachment. The macular appearance is very variable. There may be haemorrhage(s) at any layer of the retina, or a subtle grey mound (indicating subretinal neovascularization) with or without an overlying serous retinal elevation. Evidence of pre-existing pathology, in particular 'soft' drusen may be seen (**94**).

Fluorescein (and in some cases indocyanine green) angiography is often necessary to delineate the exact nature of the pathology and to assist in the decision concerning treatment (**95**).

An acute *macular hole* (see **64**) gives reduced acuity and often distortion due to a surrounding serous retinal elevation. With a 90/78D lens, a clear-cut round hole is easily seen at the fovea. With a direct ophthalmoscope, the fovea appears much more red than usual, particularly if the surrounding retina is elevated.

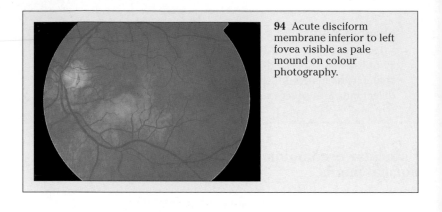

94 Acute disciform membrane inferior to left fovea visible as pale mound on colour photography.

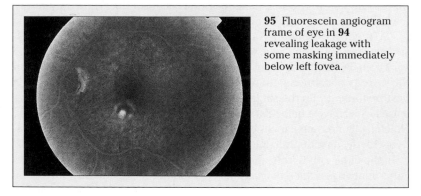

95 Fluorescein angiogram frame of eye in **94** revealing leakage with some masking immediately below left fovea.

Retinal vein occlusions usually result in blurring without distortion. A *macular branch vein occlusion* (**96**) is seen as a collection of haemorrhages, perhaps with cotton wool spots, within the vascular arcade predominantly above or below the midline. Systemic hypertension almost always is the underlying cause.

The larger *branch vein occlusions* have signs which extend outside the arcades and may reduce visual field sensitivity in the corresponding area (**97**).

Non-ischaemic *central retinal vein occlusion (CRVO)* (**98**) leads to disc oedema, dilated veins and haemorrhages with or without cotton wool spots in all four quadrants. (An afferent pupil defect in CRVO indicates significant retinal ischaemia and a risk of rubeotic [neovascular] glaucoma.) Non-ischaemic CRVO may progress to ischaemic with time.

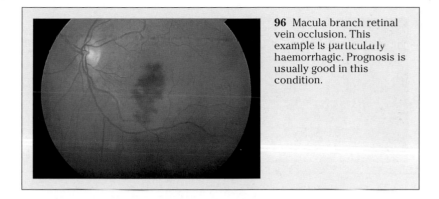

96 Macula branch retinal vein occlusion. This example is particularly haemorrhagic. Prognosis is usually good in this condition.

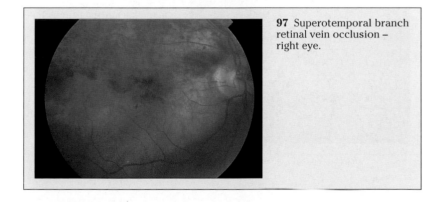

97 Superotemporal branch retinal vein occlusion – right eye.

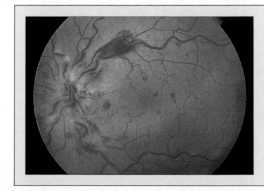

98 Central retinal vein occlusion in young patient. Note extensive disc swelling, dilated tortuous veins, blot haemorrhages extending beyond the macula. Acuity 6/6 (20/20).

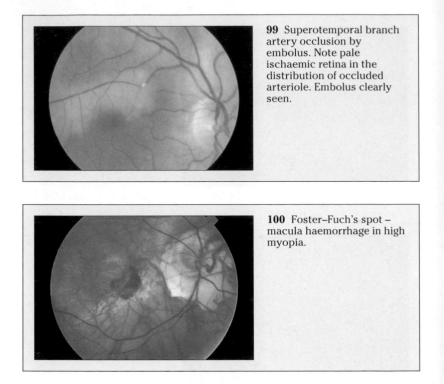

99 Superotemporal branch artery occlusion by embolus. Note pale ischaemic retina in the distribution of occluded arteriole. Embolus clearly seen.

100 Foster–Fuch's spot – macula haemorrhage in high myopia.

Small *branch arterial occlusions*, usually as a result of emboli, may reduce acuity without affecting pupil reactions, and paracentral blurring may also occur (**99**).

In high myopia, vision may rapidly deteriorate secondary to the forma-tion of a neovascular membrane under the fovea – sometimes called a *'Foster–Fuch's spot'* (**100**). Diagnosis is straightforward with an indirect viewing system, but may be difficult with direct ophthalmoscopy due to the large refractive error.

In the younger adult, aged between 20 and 50 years, a serous elevation of the macula from *central serous retinopathy* (**101**) may be difficult to detect unless it is suspected. Symptoms of acute distortion, often with micropsia and an acuity >6/18 (20/60) in a relatively featureless macula is the norm.

Rarer retinal causes of acute central visual loss include neovascular

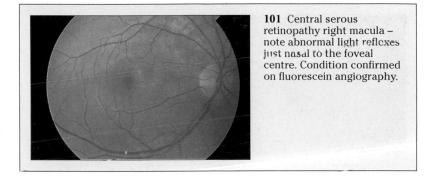

101 Central serous retinopathy right macula – note abnormal light reflexes just nasal to the foveal centre. Condition confirmed on fluorescein angiography.

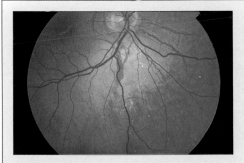

102 Angioid streaks radiating from right optic disc.

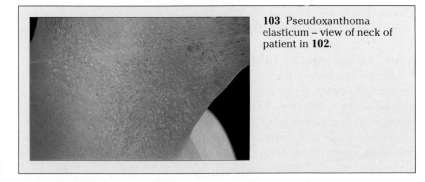

103 Pseudoxanthoma elasticum – view of neck of patient in **102**.

membrane formation in the foveal area in *angioid streaks* (**102, 103**) and *presumed ocular histoplasmosis syndrome* (**104**). In the latter, found

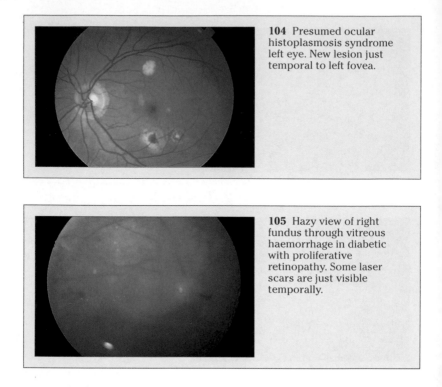

104 Presumed ocular histoplasmosis syndrome left eye. New lesion just temporal to left fovea.

105 Hazy view of right fundus through vitreous haemorrhage in diabetic with proliferative retinopathy. Some laser scars are just visible temporally.

particularly in the Midwestern US (Ohio and Mississippi River valleys), bilateral focal chorioretinal scars are seen, often with peripapillary atrophy.

Acute media opacity (RELATIVELY COMMON)

Acute *vitreous haemorrhage* (**105**) blurs vision to a degree related to its severity. If severe, there may be almost no red reflex. However, if the patient is rested sitting upright, it becomes evident on examining the red reflex, that the superior reflex is clearer than the inferior. (Direct the ophthalmoscope beam upwards while viewing from below for the superior reflex, and vice versa for the inferior.) In a less severe bleed, the use of the indirect ophthalmoscope or 90 D lens may identify the cause.

Causes of acute vitreous haemorrhage include *proliferative diabetic retinopathy* (**106**) of the macula and sickle cell retinopathy. In cases where

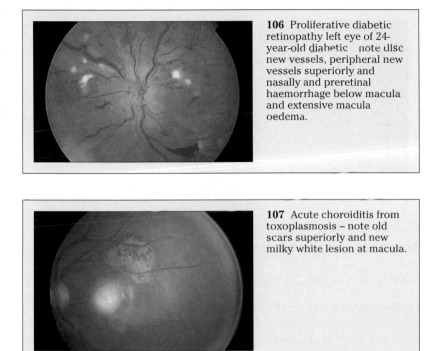

106 Proliferative diabetic retinopathy left eye of 24-year-old diabetic note disc new vessels, peripheral new vessels superiorly and nasally and preretinal haemorrhage below macula and extensive macula oedema.

107 Acute choroiditis from toxoplasmosis – note old scars superiorly and new milky white lesion at macula.

direct visualization is not possible, ultrasonography may be invaluable In determining the underlying cause. An afferent pupil defect usually indicates a coexisting retinal detachment.

Acute choroiditis (**107**) presents more slowly than vitreous haemorrhage, unless the focus of inflammation is foveal. Most cases are reactivations of old toxoplasmosis, reactivation usually occurring at the edge of an old chorioretinal scar.

Very occasionally, cataract can progress rapidly and present as acute loss of vision. A history of trauma in the past, either blunt or from an occult penetrating injury, are sought.

Spontaneous haemorrhage into the anterior chamber is VERY RARE but is easily diagnosed by the presence of hyphaema. Causes include previous blunt trauma (usually within the past 10 days), Fuch's heterochromic cyclitis, and iris lesions.

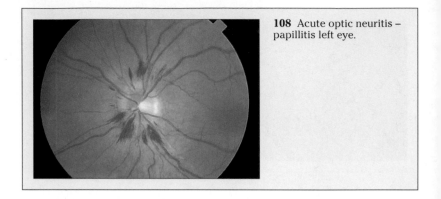

108 Acute optic neuritis – papillitis left eye.

Uniocular predominantly central visual loss: abnormal pupil reaction

In the presence of an afferent pupil defect, other diagnoses are more likely.

Optic nerve disease (COMMON)

In the younger adult, *optic neuritis* (**108**) or *retrobulbar neuritis* must be excluded. Decreased sensitivity to red targets and an afferent pupil defect are usually present. The acuity may be at any level from 6/6 (20/20) to NLP. In the former, a papillitis is observed, but in the first few weeks of the latter the optic disc often looks normal. In the latter, pain on ocular movement is common. Previous history of neurological symptoms increases the likelihood of multiple sclerosis as the cause and the fellow eye may demonstrate subtle temporal optic atrophy from a previous subclinical attack.

In the older adult, an *ischaemic optic neuropathy* (**109**) is a common cause of sudden uniocular visual loss. The disc usually appears pale and swollen, often with small haemorrhages at its margin. An altitudinal field defect commonly coexists as either the upper or lower disc may be affected. *Cranial arteritis* (**110**) must always be excluded, although diabetes and hypertension are often implicated in non-vasculitic cases. Acuity may vary from 6/6 (20/20) to NLP, and is not a guide to the presence of vasculitis.

Retinal disease (COMMON)

In *central retinal artery occlusion* (**111**), the history is acute, the vision is very poor (HM or LP) and, in the early stages, the retina looks milky white

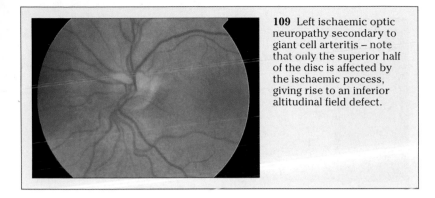

109 Left ischaemic optic neuropathy secondary to giant cell arteritis – note that only the superior half of the disc is affected by the ischaemic process, giving rise to an inferior altitudinal field defect.

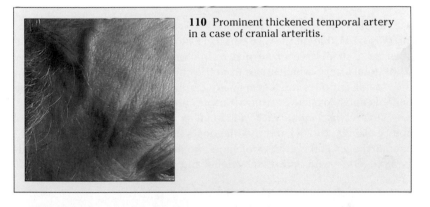

110 Prominent thickened temporal artery in a case of cranial arteritis.

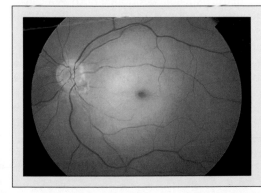

111 Central retinal artery occlusion left eye, in this case secondary to hypertension – note the cherry-red spot at the fovea.

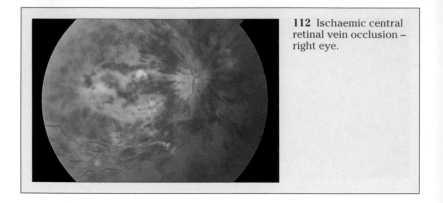

112 Ischaemic central retinal vein occlusion – right eye.

with a 'cherry red spot' at the fovea due to ganglion cell oedema. An embolus may be visible on the disc surface. Cilioretinal artery sparing may be seen as a small area of normal retina surrounded by oedema. If the cilioretinal artery, which arises from the choroidal circulation rather than the retinal, supplies the fovea, acuity can be normal! As time passes, the oedema subsides, leaving thin arterioles and optic atrophy.

A severely *ischaemic CRVO* (**112**) gives an afferent pupil defect, poor acuity (<6/60 [20/20]) and the diagnosis is straightforward as multiple haemorrhages and cotton wool spots are present in all four retinal quadrants together with optic disc oedema and dilated, tortuous veins.

Adie's syndrome (RARE)
This cause of uniocular visual disturbance is mentioned here as a cause of reduced near vision in the younger adult. The ciliary ganglion is the site of damage in what is presumed to be a post-viral 'mononeuritis'. Typically the patient notices blurred reading vision (and distance if hypermetropic) and some degree of dazzling in bright light. Some notice the enlarged pupil on the side of the lesion. Visual acuity is normal with a pinhole and the pupil reacts slowly to light (**113**), and is slow to dilate following constriction (tonic pupil). Established cases show light-near dissociation and denervation hypersensitivity to 0.125% pilocarpine (normal pupils do not constrict to this concentration). On slit lamp examination, characteristic writhing movements of the iris are seen with segmental contraction of the sphincter.

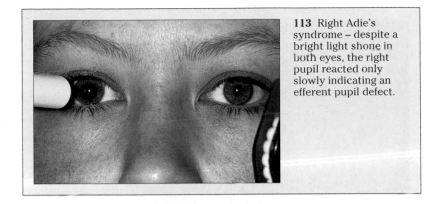

113 Right Adie's syndrome – despite a bright light shone in both eyes, the right pupil reacted only slowly indicating an efferent pupil defect.

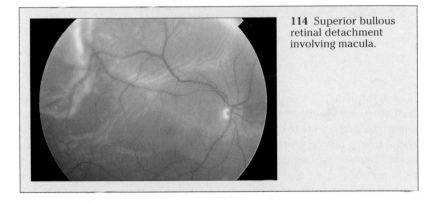

114 Superior bullous retinal detachment involving macula.

Acute uniocular peripheral visual loss (RELATIVELY COMMON)

Beware the patient who notices a pre-existing pathology and relates the symptoms as acute. Always consider chronic causes of peripheral field loss here (see Chapter 4).

Acute rhegmatogenous retinal detachment causes a total field loss consistent with the extent of retinal separation (**114**). As a result of the anatomy, the field defect does not respect either the horizontal or vertical meridians and, in the absence of significant vitreous haemorrhage, acuity is usually

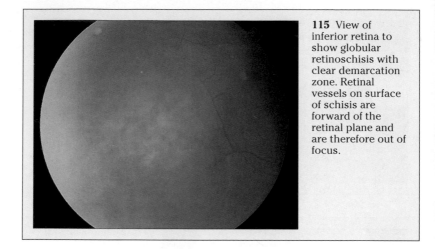

115 View of inferior retina to show globular retinoschisis with clear demarcation zone. Retinal vessels on surface of schisis are forward of the retinal plane and are therefore out of focus.

normal if the macula remains attached. The detached retina can be visualized when viewing the red reflex as a billowing sheet with thin vessels superimposed. Indirect ophthalmoscopy usually determines the position of the retinal tear(s) and/or hole(s) that lead to the detachment. Superior detachments may progress very rapidly, particularly if the breaks are large or in aphakia, and only a small segment of retina may remain attached. Inferior detachments may progress slowly and retinal pigment lines can delineate rising levels of subretinal fluid. Occasionally *retinoschisis*, which also causes loss of peripheral vision, presents (**115**). This relatively static globular retinal 'cyst' is often bilateral and inferotemporally sited. Differentiation from a slowly progressive rhegmatogenous detachment may be difficult, requiring sequential examinations over time.

Other causes of acute significant monocular peripheral field defects are rare but retinal migraine must be considered in a susceptible individual with a typical history of a field defect persisting after a monocular attack. *Ischaemic optic neuropathy, retinal branch artery occlusion, optic nerve head drusen* (see **82**) are also rare causes, as is *cytomegalovirus retinitis* (usually in an HIV-positive individual) where peripheral disease may cause symptoms (**116**).

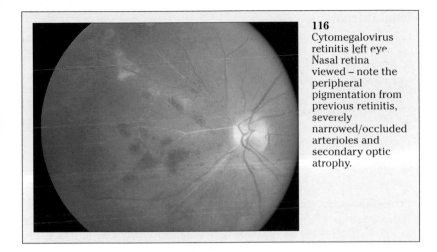

116
Cytomegalovirus retinitis left eye. Nasal retina viewed – note the peripheral pigmentation from previous retinitis, severely narrowed/occluded arterioles and secondary optic atrophy.

Uniocular acute visual disturbances (COMMON)

These may take the form of:
- Amaurosis fugax, where visual function, usually involving acuity, is disturbed temporarily but with full recovery.
- Visual intrusions, where abnormal visual stimulations occur. These may be constant or intermittent, but visual function remains unchanged.

Amaurosis fugax
A history of intermittent loss of visual function lasting less than 1 hour followed by full recovery prompts the examiner to look for clues as to its cause. Often, no clues are found on ophthalmic examination, but the likely cause can be determined due to the physical status of the patient. This is particularly true in amaurosis fugax from retinal emboli, where small cholesterol deposits may be seen in the retinal arterioles. Carotid and/or cardiac signs are sought by clinical examination and/or ultrasonography.

Other causes of uniocular amaurosis include cranial arteritis, optic nerve head drusen, and dysthyroid disease.

Visual intrusions

> ### Strategy point
> Examine the vitreous carefully for cells, pigment and for the presence of a visible posterior vitreous face. (Tilt a horizontal slit lamp beam upwards slightly and focus deep in the vitreous cavity to see a posterior vitreous detachment (PVD). A 'membrane' beyond which is an optically clear space is seen in a PVD.)

The most common visual intrusion is from 'benign floaters'. These minor opacities in the vitreous are visible to many normal individuals (usually in both eyes) as they become older when viewing a light background. Myopes are particularly troubled by benign floaters.

A sudden shower of floaters indicates the possibility of vitreous haemorrhage. Careful examination of the peripheral retina is necessary to exclude a retinal break as the cause of the symptoms. This can only be performed adequately with an indirect ophthalmoscope and/or a contact lens examination with a slit lamp as the break may be very peripherally sited. The absence of cells or pigment in the vitreous lowers the likelihood of associated retinal pathology significantly.

The appearance of a single formed floater, often in the shape of a ring, is usually due to a posterior vitreous detachment, an event that occurs in most eyes by the age of 75 years of age. It is often accompanied by a period of intermittent flashing lights, usually most obvious to the patient in dim lighting. Again, a retinal tear must be excluded. (Flashes occurring in brighter lighting conditions increase the probability of a coexisting retinal tear.)

Monocular flickering light, usually in the periphery, always prompts a retinal examination as expanding lesions such as *malignant melanoma* (see **72**) may present in this way.

Entoptic phenomena (physiological visual intrusions manifest under certain circumstances) may present for exclusion. Benign floaters are so common as to be included in this category. Other phenomena include the perception of one's retinal vessels (and sometimes white blood cells) when a blue light is shone in the eye from a certain angle and the small semicircular paracentral flashes of light produced by rapid movement of the eyes in the dark-adapted state (phosphenes).

Monocular diplopia

Alteration of refractive error (COMMON)

The most common cause of monocular diplopia is *early cataract* (see 55–57) which may also give polyopia (multiple images). This may be intermittent depending on lighting conditions.

External pressure on the eye such as from a large *chalazion* (see **169**) on the upper lid, may give rise to a rapid onset induced astigmatism and 'ghosting', reported as 'double vision' by the patient. A pinhole relieves the 'diplopia', confirming the refractive nature of the problem

Binocular acute central visual loss

> **Strategy point**
> Take care to note the pupils here, significant visual loss with normal pupils and retinal examination indicates either cortical blindness or hysteria/malingering.

Retinal causes (RARE)

Cytomegalovirus retinitis (see **116**) may cause bilateral severe acute loss of vision, retinal signs being described as 'like a tomato and cheese pizza'.

In acute multifocal placoid pigment epitheliopathy (AMPPE), multiple small raised lesions are present at both maculae in a young patient in whom a history of recent respiratory infection is common. Acuities are usually >6/24 (20/80) with subtotal recovery being the norm.

Acute rises in blood pressure may induce macular oedema. This may occur in pregnancy (toxaemia) or from *phaeochromocytoma* (**117**).

In acute quinine poisoning, vision is reduced from retinal arterial spasm.

Optic nerve causes (RARE)

In bilateral *optic neuritis* similar signs are seen to those found in the uniocular condition. Pure bilateral simultaneous disease is rare in multiple sclerosis and suggests an alternative diagnosis such as *infiltrative ophthalmopathy* (see **43**) (e.g. from leukaemia or sarcoidosis) in younger patients or *ischaemic optic neuropathy* in older adults (**118**).

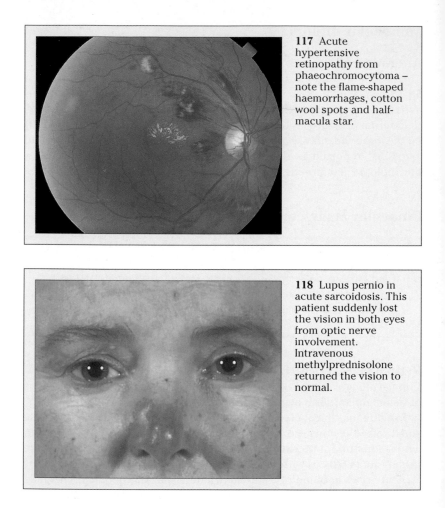

117 Acute hypertensive retinopathy from phaeochromocytoma – note the flame-shaped haemorrhages, cotton wool spots and half-macula star.

118 Lupus pernio in acute sarcoidosis. This patient suddenly lost the vision in both eyes from optic nerve involvement. Intravenous methylprednisolone returned the vision to normal.

In *chronic papilloedema* (**119**), typically as a result of benign intracranial hypertension, acute decompensation of the optic nerve head may occur leading to bilateral visual loss. The grossly swollen optic discs with a champagne cork appearance must not be confused with optic neuritis where a more gradual slope is seen at the disc edge. (Mild papilloedema does not usually cause visual symptoms.)

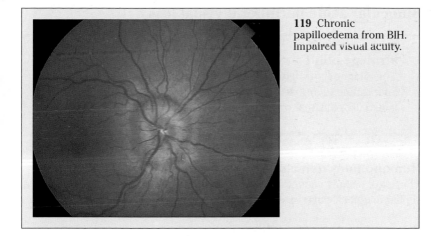

119 Chronic papilloedema from BIH. Impaired visual acuity.

Cortical causes (RARE)

Central scotomas of acute onset may be as a result of recent cortical disease, either infarction or haemorrhage into a tumour. Pupils are normal, as is ophthalmoscopy. Peripheral fields may also be affected (see Chapter 4).

Strategy point

Think of hysteria/malingering in a young patient whose symptoms do not fit with the signs.

In hysterical visual loss, visual function may be recorded at any level but it is usually <6/24 (20/80). Letters are read slowly – even with larger print – than the best level recorded. Additional lines may be seen with persuasion, particularly with cancelling lenses in the trial frame. Visual fields may be 'cylindrical' (same size for different targets or at different working distances) or 'spiral' (progressively smaller during the test) when recorded on the Bjerrum screen or a perimeter. Malingering patients have 'insight' and usually have something to gain, often financially, from their apparent loss of vision, whereas hysterical individuals may be in need of counselling or psychiatric help. Monocular hysteria/malingering also occurs.

Binocular acute peripheral visual loss

Strategy point
The diagnosis is usually evident following testing the fields. Spend time identifying the exact field defect. In the acute case it is usually chiasmal or retrochiasmal.

Homonomous defects – (retrochiasmal) (COMMON)
These are usually caused by a stroke, although tumours may present in a similar manner. Ocular examination only rarely contributes to the diagnosis.

Bitemporal defects – (chiasmal)
If they present acutely, bitemporal defects are usually severe. In younger patients the differential diagnosis is between acute demyelination of the chiasm, almost always as part of multiple sclerosis, and acute chiasmal compression. Some degree of central visual loss is common, if only loss of colour and contrast, but acuity measured by Snellen or similar may be 'normal'. Temporal optic atrophy at presentation may indicate that the disease process has been present for longer than the symptoms would suggest and makes compression the more likely diagnosis.

Bilateral defects not restricted by meridia
These are RARE, and bilateral physical signs corresponding to the field defects are sought. The following is not an exhaustive list but serves to illustrate the mental process required: retinal detachment; secondary choroidal tumours; optic nerve head drusen; and cytomegalovirus retinitis.

Binocular acute visual disturbances (COMMON)

Strategy point
Establish from the history whether diplopia is present.

Without diplopia

These include the entoptic phenomena described under monocular disturbances.

The most common 'pathological' manifestation is during a migraine attack, where the visual disturbance can range from a mild peripheral shimmering, to incapacitating central scotomata. The history and full recovery are suggestive of the diagnosis, but visual symptoms often occur in previously non-migranous subjects over the age of 40 years, without other phenomena typical of the condition such as aura and headache.

Very occasionally a hemianopia may persist as a result of permanent damage to the visual pathways.

Raised intracranial pressure may present with intermittent bilateral obscurations of vision. These often occur when coughing, straining or when rising from a seated position and may result from optic nerve or cortical malfunction. Papilloedema is invariably present in both eyes.

With diplopia

Strategy point

Ensure that the diplopia is binocular. Patients often do not appreciate that double vision can be present in one eye!

Strategy point

Is the diplopia intermittent or constant, horizontal, vertical or mixed, and in which position of gaze is it at its worst? Quickly check the visual fields as severe bilateral field defects close to fixation may induce diplopia. Now look for a compensatory head tilt and check the extraocular movements.

Acute diplopia may be due to disease of the central control systems, the cranial nerves (III, IV and VI) or the extraocular muscles themselves. Look for a recognisable pattern. Think *myaesthenia* (**120**) or dysthyroid if a classical pattern is absent.

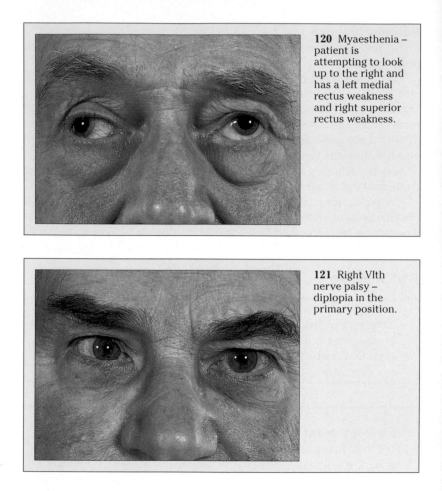

120 Myaesthenia – patient is attempting to look up to the right and has a left medial rectus weakness and right superior rectus weakness.

121 Right VIth nerve palsy – diplopia in the primary position.

Horizontal diplopia
Sixth nerve palsy (COMMON)
A pure horizontal diplopia maximal with gaze to the side of the lesion is seen (**121**). Head turn towards the side of the lesion is common if subtotal or in a recovery phase. Unilateral VIth nerve palsies are often secondary to diabetes or idiopathic. Bilateral involvement suggests raised intracranial pressure or brain stem disease. The clinical condition will determine the appropriate course of action.

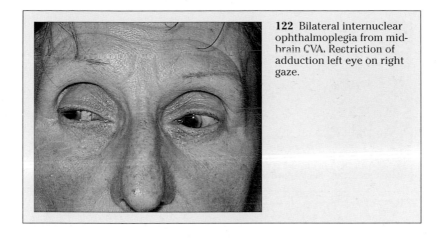

122 Bilateral internuclear ophthalmoplegia from midbrain CVA. Restriction of adduction left eye on right gaze.

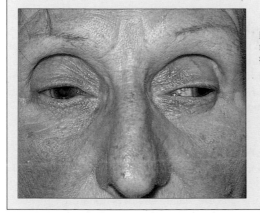

123 Same patient as in **122**, looking left. Restriction of adduction right eye – partial WEBINO syndrome.

Brain stem disease (RARE)

In an *internuclear ophthalmoplegia* there is failure of adduction on the side of the lesion with nystagmoid movements of the abducting eye (**122**). This may be bilateral with a divergent squint in the primary position (WEBINO) syndrome; **123**. In a 'one-and-a-half' syndrome, an internuclear ophthalmoplegia coexists with a gaze palsy, so the only horizontal movement is abduction of one eye with nystagmus.

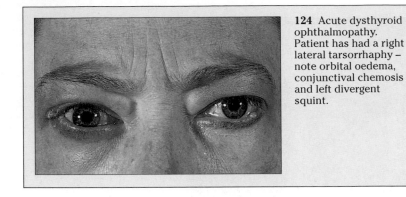

124 Acute dysthyroid ophthalmopathy. Patient has had a right lateral tarsorrhaphy – note orbital oedema, conjunctival chemosis and left divergent squint.

Restrictive ophthalmopathy (RARE)

This may simulate a VIth with the medial rectus involved, or a medial rectus weakness with the lateral rectus involved. In the developmental anomaly termed Duane's retraction syndrome, there is a weakness of abduction, combined with retraction of the globe and narrowing of the palpebral aperture on adduction, which may also be weak.

Vertical diplopia

Restrictive ophthalmopathy (COMMON)

Dysthyroid disease usually causes a limitation of elevation in one or both eyes, usually asymmetrically, from fibrosis of the inferior rectus muscle(s) (**124**). The associated proptosis aids the diagnosis but is not always present. A blow-out fracture of the orbit is suggested by the history of trauma, a relative enophthalmos, hypothesia in areas supplied by branches of the maxillary division of the trigeminal, and usually a restriction of upgaze.

IVth nerve palsy (COMMON)

A head tilt is often seen (**125**). The separation of images is maximal looking down away from the side of the lesion, and a tilted image is common in acute cases. It is not uncommon for decompensated long-standing cases to present as 'acute'. Ask for a history of head trauma in the past and expect a compensatory head posture and less tilt on the images.

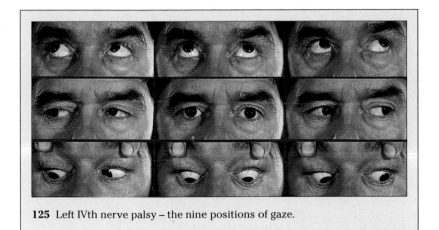

125 Left IVth nerve palsy – the nine positions of gaze.

Vertical gaze palsy (RARE)

Occasionally, dorsal midbrain syndrome (Parinaud's) causes vertical diplopia. Downgaze and horizontal movements are intact. Attempted upgaze produces a subtle retraction of the globes, emphasized with an optokinetic drum rotating slowly downwards (to induce upward saccades). Light/near dissociation of the pupils may be demonstrable from the lesion in the pretectal area at the level of the superior colliculus.

Mixed horizontal and vertical diplopia

IIIrd nerve palsy (RARE)

The diagnosis is usually straightforward as a number of extraocular muscles are involved and a ptosis is often present (**126, 127**). Those with the pupil affected (dilated) are much more likely to be secondary to compressive lesions such as posterior communicating artery aneurysm.

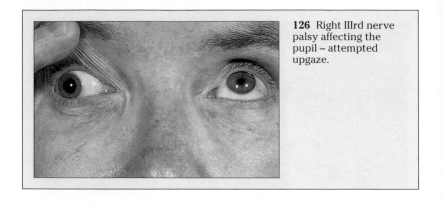

126 Right IIIrd nerve palsy affecting the pupil – attempted upgaze.

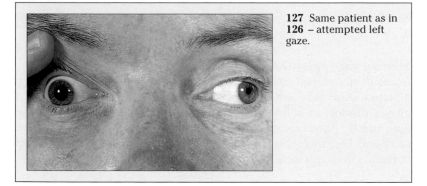

127 Same patient as in **126** – attempted left gaze.

Strategy point

Check for a coexisting IVth by asking the patient to look down to the side opposite the lesion. If the top of the eye rotates inwards (look at the conjunctival blood vessels at the superior limbus), the IVth is intact. Check for a Vth (including corneal sensation) and a VIth in the usual way – combined palsies are usually due to cavernous sinus or orbital apex disease.

CHAPTER 6

THE ACUTE RED EYE

The acute red eye				
Uniocular				
No Pain	**Pain**			
	Vision normal		**Vision reduced**	
Vision normal	Corneal Staining?			
	No	Yes	No	Yes
Subconjunctival haemorrhage Episcleritis Pterygium Pingueculum Conjunctivitis	Anterior uveitis Scleritis HZO (early)	Herpes simplex Marginal ulcer	Severe uveitis Angle closure glaucoma Secondary glaucoma	Herpes simplex Bacterial keratitis HZO
Binocular				
No pain/good vision		**Pain/vision good or poor**		
Bacterial conjunctivitis Viral conjunctivitis Allergic conjunctivitis		Viral keratoconjunctivitis Chlamydial keratoconjunctivitis Vernal catarrh Arc eye		

This chapter covers conditions varying from the most commonly encountered ocular problems with minimal morbidity to rarer, sight-threatening disorders. Distinguishing between the two requires care and a constant mental note to oneself that all red eyes are not necessarily conjunctivitis. Chronic irritations and redness are considered in Chapter 8, but an acute exacerbation of a chronic condition must be kept in mind when diagnosing acute red eyes. When lists of conditions are given under a subheading, the most common are always given first, with the least common last.

Strategy point – the History

Ascertain first any history of trauma, contact lens use or previous surgery as these special cases are discussed in their own subsections. Any ocular self-medication is noted, as sensitivity to such agents must be excluded. Patients can now be divided into subgroups based upon the answers to three important questions:

1. Is it one eye or both?
2. Is it painful or sensitive to light rather than uncomfortable?
3. Is your vision blurred to an extent that it doesn't clear on blinking?

Accurate answers to these questions narrow down the probabilities significantly.

Strategy point

Measure the acuities in each eye and inspect the anterior segments carefully, noting any lid or facial abnormalities (lid conditions giving rise to red eyes are considered in Chapter 7). If the answer to either of questions 2 and 3 above is positive, fluorescein dye is used to determine if any corneal staining is present.

One eye, no pain and good vision

If the redness is focal, the diagnosis is likely to be between spontaneous subconjunctival haemorrhage, episcleritis, and inflamed pingueculum/pterygium.

In *spontaneous subconjunctival haemorrhage*, (COMMON) a brick-red, well-defined area is seen, obscuring the vessels of the conjunctiva (**128**).

In *episcleritis* (COMMON) there is a focal dilation of conjunctival and episcleral vessels, usually adjacent to the limbus (**129**). A small nodule may be present and irritation rather than pain occurs.

Raised lesions of the conjunctiva (COMMON) may cause irritation and focal redness from their physical presence disrupting the tear film. The most common are pingueculae and *pterygia* (**130**), but *papillomata*

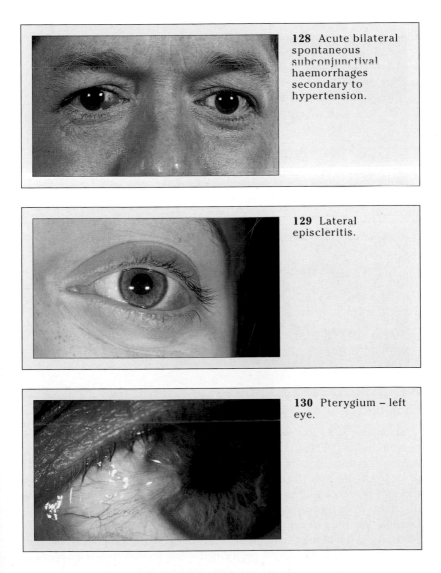

128 Acute bilateral spontaneous subconjunctival haemorrhages secondary to hypertension.

129 Lateral episcleritis.

130 Pterygium – left eye.

occasionally arise from the caruncle or tarsal conjunctiva as red glutinous masses (**131**). (Malignant lesions are considered if the appearance and/or site of a lesion is atypical.)

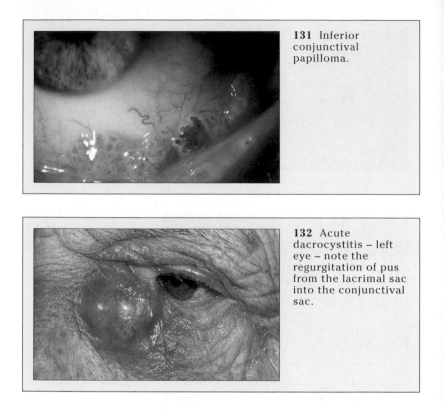

131 Inferior conjunctival papilloma.

132 Acute dacrocystitis – left eye – note the regurgitation of pus from the lacrimal sac into the conjunctival sac.

Stickiness and a more diffuse redness would suggest a form of infective conjunctivitis (VERY COMMON) in its early stages (before bilaterality). Always consider chronic reinfection from an occluded nasolacrimal duct in recurrent disease. The duct is not patent on syringing and pressure over the medial canthal area may result in regurgitation of creamy yellow discharge from the lower punctum. Occasionally, the chronically infected lacrimal sac may develop acute inflammation – an *acute dacrocystitis* (**132**). A search along the lid margin for the typical lesions of *molluscum contagiosum* (**133**) (RARE) is performed when a single eye with chronic conjunctivitis does not respond to the usual antibiotics.

Chronically dilated blood vessels with an unusual appearance may indicate rarer conditions such as *caroticocavernous sinus fistula* (see **182, 183**), hereditary haemorrhagic telangectasia, or sickle cell disease.

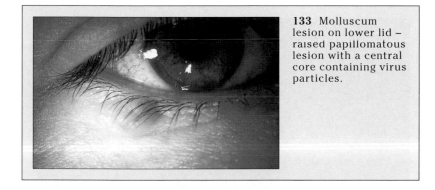

133 Molluscum lesion on lower lid – raised papillomatous lesion with a central core containing virus particles.

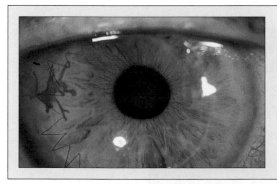

134 Herpes simplex dendrite stained with Rose Bengal in an eye with recent penetrating keratoplasty (corneal transplant).

One eye, pain but good vision

Strategy point
Pain and/or photophobia indicates intraocular or significant ocular coat inflammation/infection or markedly raised intraocular pressure (IOP), not just 'conjunctivitis'.

With corneal staining
The branching 'dendrite' from *herpes simplex keratitis* (COMMON) is pathognomonic (**134**). Lesions off the visual axis are compatible with normal acuity.

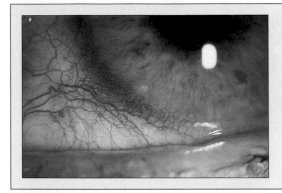

135 Marginal corneal ulcer – unstained – small lesion (almost in centre of slide) with the associated limbal injection. Note irregular lid margin from staphylococcal lid disease.

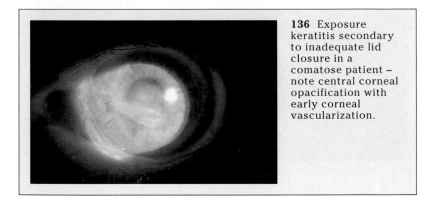

136 Exposure keratitis secondary to inadequate lid closure in a comatose patient – note central corneal opacification with early corneal vascularization.

Marginal ulceration (**135**) (COMMON) is usually accompanied by focal conjunctival/episcleral injection. Blepharitis (often bilateral) may lead to these ulcers which occur as a result of a hypersensitivity to bacterial proteins (see **204, 205**).

An 'inferior third' staining area on the cornea suggests *exposure keratitis* from lagophthalmos (**136**), and lid closure is tested, paying attention to the presence or absence of Bell's phenomenon.

A 'gutter' ulcer running circumferentially around the corneal periphery with staining indicates active corneal melting and may arise as a result of collagen disease such as rheumatoid disease or the very rare *Mooren's ulcer* (**137**).

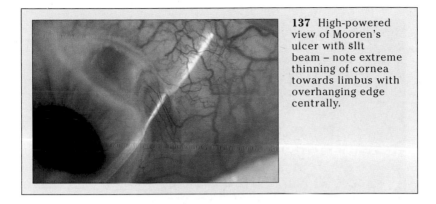

137 High-powered view of Mooren's ulcer with slit beam – note extreme thinning of cornea towards limbus with overhanging edge centrally.

Strategy point
Take care to exclude lid conditions such as entropion and trichiasis if the staining pattern suggests recurrent trauma to the cornea (see Chapter 7).

Without corneal staining

Circumlimbal redness and a small pupil suggests *anterior uveitis (iritis)* (COMMON). Photophobia and pain on accommodation are common, most patients being young adults if it is their first attack, and a positive history of HLA B27 disease may be obtained. Slit lamp examination reveals cells and flare in the AC and keratic precipitates (KPs) may be seen, sited maximally on the inferior endothelium (**138**). Posterior synechiae may be visible.

Focal scleral redness with a dull, aching pain suggests *scleritis* (RARE), which may be nodular, diffuse or necrotizing (**139**). Some conjunctival staining over the lesion may be seen and if extensive suggests the necrotizing variety. Episcleritis 'blanches' with 0.1% adrenaline whereas the deep inflammation of scleritis does not. Scleritis is also usually tender to gentle touch through the closed eyelid and a bluish colour may be seen in natural light.

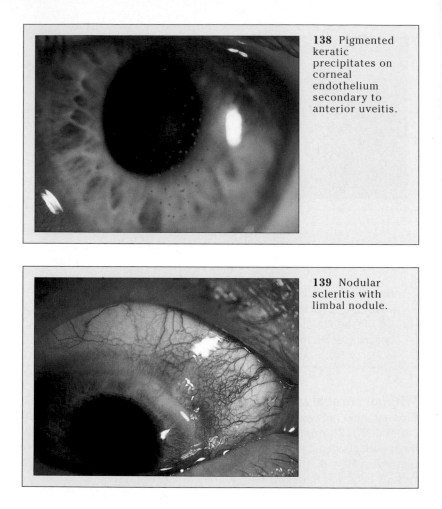

138 Pigmented keratic precipitates on corneal endothelium secondary to anterior uveitis.

139 Nodular scleritis with limbal nodule.

A uniocular watery conjunctivitis with pain out of proportion to the signs raises the possibility of *herpes zoster ophthalmicus (HZO)* (UNCOMMON) (see **199**). There may be few, if any, skin vesicles in the early stages, or they may be hidden above the hair line. Vesicles may occur in the distribution of the external nasal division of the ophthalmic branch of the trigeminal, on the side of the nose, towards its tip.

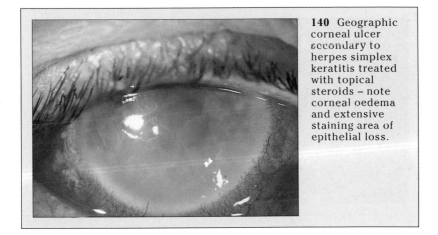

140 Geographic corneal ulcer secondary to herpes simplex keratitis treated with topical steroids – note corneal oedema and extensive staining area of epithelial loss.

One eye, pain and reduced vision

More severe cases of those diagnoses mentioned in the preceding section may cause visual loss in proportion to their severity. With intraocular and/or corneal inflammation, conjunctival injection is maximal around the limbus.

With corneal staining

A *herpes simplex dendritic ulcer* (COMMON) on the visual axis reduces vision. Inappropriate treatment of a dendritic ulcer with topical steroids produces a *geographic ulcer* (**140**) and may result in corneal perforation.

Acute keratitis (RARE) from bacteria and fungi results in a centrally staining ulcer surrounded by opacity from abscess formation and/or corneal stromal oedema (**141**). A hypopyon may be present and the eye is usually sticky from purulent exudation. Penetration into the cornea by bacteria and fungi is rare in the absence of trauma or immunodeficiency; however, the patient may not have been aware of the precipitating incident.

Established HZO (UNCOMMON) results in diffuse superficial punctate staining or microdendrites on slit lamp examination. Vision may be reduced from these corneal epithelial disturbances, stromal oedema with or without raised IOP, or, more rarely, retinal or optic nerve involvement.

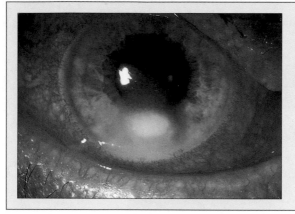

141 Acute bacterial keratitis – note focus of infection just inferior to centre of cornea, inferior corneal oedema and early vascular response into cornea inferiorly.

Without corneal staining

The following causes are all UNCOMMON.

Anterior uveitis with significant secondary corneal oedema from extensive KPs and/or raised IOP reduces vision. An important but rare variant is sympathetic ophthalmia. In this condition a spontaneous granulomatous uveitis occurs in the fellow eye of an eye which has suffered trauma (usually penetrating) in the past. Both anterior and posterior uveitis occur and either may predominate. If the latter, yellowish spots may be seen in the retina (Dalen–Fuch's nodules) through the vitritis.

Conjunctival injection, maximal in the circumlimbal position in association with corneal oedema and a fixed mid-dilated pupil suggests *acute angle closure glaucoma (AACG)* (**142**) or *rubeotic glaucoma* (**143**). In both the acuity is very poor at CF, HM or LP, the IOP is markedly raised on digital or applanation tonometry and the patient may be systemically unwell with nausea/vomiting. In the former, a history of attacks aborted by sleep may be helpful, but most patients present with their first attack.

In AACG, many patients are hypermetropic to a significant degree (examine the distance spectacles – they magnify print) and the fellow eye has a narrow angle (best demonstrated on gonioscopy with a slit lamp).

A history of profound visual loss (from CRVO) in the weeks preceding the attack or of diabetic retinopathy suggests rubeotic glaucoma, as does the finding of rubeotic vessels on the iris. These may be difficult to see due to the corneal oedema – even with the slit lamp – and a lightly

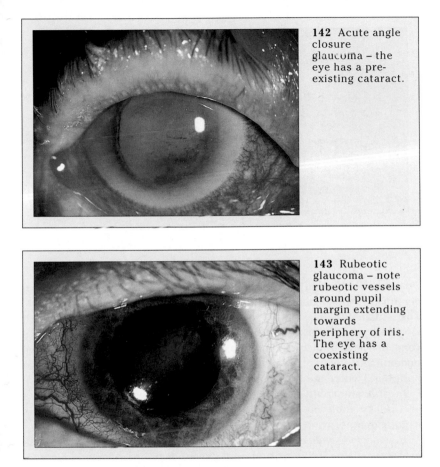

142 Acute angle closure glaucoma – the eye has a pre-existing cataract.

143 Rubeotic glaucoma – note rubeotic vessels around pupil margin extending towards periphery of iris. The eye has a coexisting cataract.

coloured iris may display dilated vessels in AACG. Reducing the oedema with systemic or topical ocular antihypertensives and/or topical glycerol or methylcellulose may improve the view and enable an accurate diagnosis.

Raised IOP with corneal oedema is also found in anterior uveitis from secondary dysfunction of the trabecular meshwork. Although the uveitis is usually marked, sometimes a significantly raised IOP occurs with minimal inflammation, the Posner–Schlossman syndrome. A single (sentinel) KP may be seen through the corneal oedema and the pupil is small.

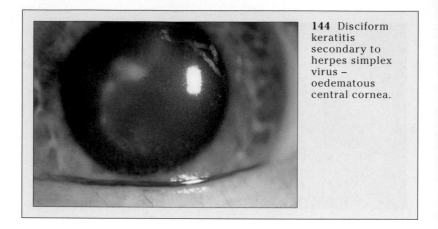

144 Disciform keratitis secondary to herpes simplex virus – oedematous central cornea.

A specific type of reaction to the herpes simplex virus – *disciform keratitis* – results in a central non-staining corneal opacity (**144**).
The remaining causes in this section are RARE.

A 360° posterior synechiae may cause a secondary angle closure glaucoma in uveitis from 'iris bombe'. A small pupil is seen through the corneal oedema and the central anterior chamber is usually deep – unlike the peripheral where the iris is in contact with the cornea.

In phacomorphic glaucoma, a cataractous swollen lens causes a secondary angle closure. The central AC is shallow and the lens is usually opaque.

In *phacolytic glaucoma* (**145**) a mature cataractous lens begins to leak protein, causing inflammation and a secondary open angle glaucoma. Amorphous lens material is usually present in the AC which is deep.

In the very rare metastatic endophthalmitis, a hypopyon is combined with vitreous opacity. A history of drug abuse or HIV-positive status (*Candida* endophthalmitis) or septic foci elsewhere in the body aids the diagnosis.

The above conditions usually do not cause significant lid swelling. If seen, *preseptal cellulitis* (see **35**) and *orbital cellulitis* (**146**) are considered, particularly in children where a history of recent upper respiratory tract infection is common. In preseptal cellulitis, ocular movements and vision are good and a source of infection may be seen on the lids. However in

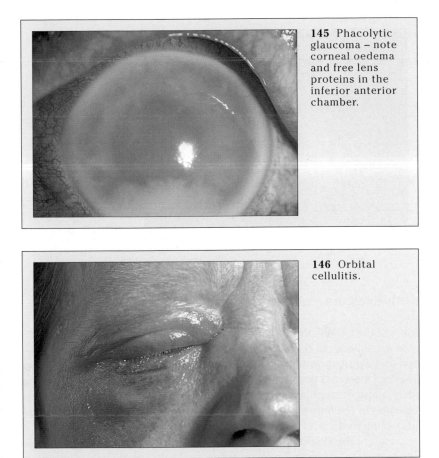

145 Phacolytic glaucoma – note corneal oedema and free lens proteins in the inferior anterior chamber.

146 Orbital cellulitis.

orbital cellulitis, proptosis and restricted ocular movements are seen and vision may be markedly reduced.

Although usually a neonatal condition, acute gonococcal conjunctivitis may occur in adults from autoinnoculation from infected genitalia. A rapid-onset, painful purulent conjunctivitis with lid swelling is seen. Delayed treatment may lead to corneal ulceration and rapid perforation as the organism can penetrate the intact epithelium.

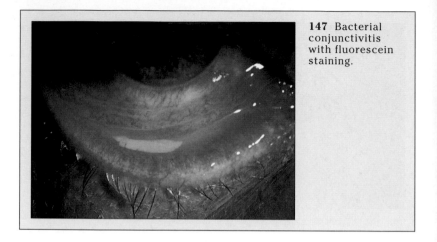

147 Bacterial conjunctivitis with fluorescein staining.

Both eyes, no pain and good vision

Some of the COMMONEST conditions of the eye occur in this section.

In *acute bacterial conjunctivitis* (**147**) there is diffuse conjunctival injection and a mucopurulent discharge causing the lids to stick together on waking. One eye is usually symptomatic a day or so before its fellow, but early signs of papillae and redness of the tarsal conjunctiva can be detected in the fellow eye. Follicles (see below) do not occur in bacterial conjunctivitis.

Uncomplicated *viral conjunctivitis* may be preceded by an upper respiratory tract infection and may be associated with a vesicular eruption on the face (primary HSV and adenovirus), especially around the eyes (**148**). Follicles may be seen in the inferior fornix as dome-shaped elevations with a pale centre, and small subconjunctival haemorrhages are seen with certain viruses (enterovirus, Epstein–Barr). The plica and caruncle can often become hyperaemic, particularly in adenovirus disease. A palpable preauricular gland is a non-specific sign.

Acute *allergic conjunctivitis* (**149**) presents seasonally in temperate climates. In 'hay fever conjunctivitis' the main symptom is itching, which can be severe. Diffuse redness of the conjunctiva is present with a watery

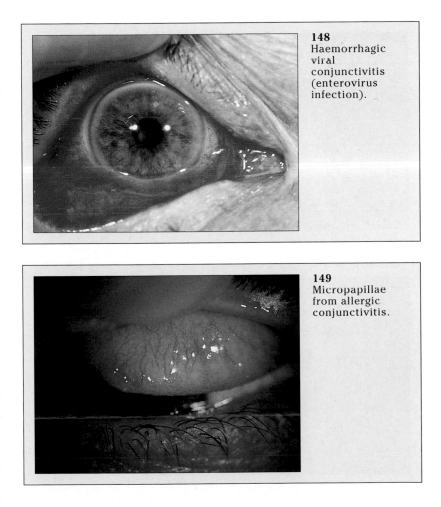

148
Haemorrhagic
viral
conjunctivitis
(enterovirus
infection).

149
Micropapillae
from allergic
conjunctivitis.

discharge, sometimes with stringy mucus which accumulates in the medial canthus (**150**). In season, symptoms are brought on by exposure to allergen, and are often associated with nasal irritation and itching of the palate. Occasionally, acute conjunctival chemosis occurs following exposure to large volumes of allergen.

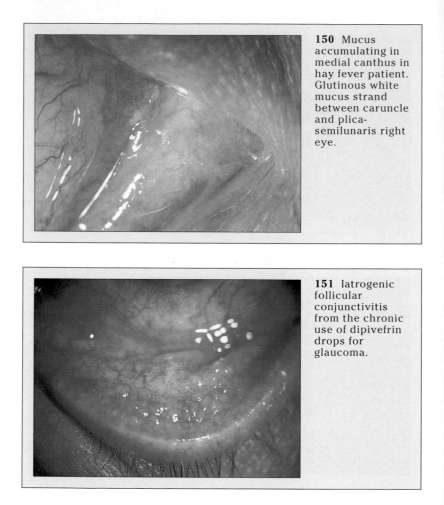

150 Mucus accumulating in medial canthus in hay fever patient. Glutinous white mucus strand between caruncle and plica-semilunaris right eye.

151 Iatrogenic follicular conjunctivitis from the chronic use of dipivefrin drops for glaucoma.

Iatrogenic conjunctivitis is common with certain antiglaucoma agents, particularly dipivefrin, where a pronounced follicular reaction is seen (**151**). Agents containing adrenaline often cause a rebound diffuse hyperaemia, and adenochrome deposits appearing as black dots in the inferior fornix may be seen.

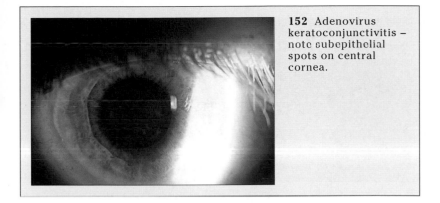

152 Adenovirus keratoconjunctivitis – note subepithelial spots on central cornea.

Both eyes, pain, with or without vision affected

Viral keratoconjunctivitis (UNCOMMON) gives photophobia which may be severe (**152**). Although acuity may be reduced, it is usually normal or almost normal. The most common virus to induce a bilateral keratitis is the adenovirus type 8. As well as the signs in the conjunctiva outlined above, multiple superficial opacities are visible in the cornea which stain in the early phase of the disease. Epithelial punctate lesions with variable superficial stromal involvement are seen with the slit lamp, together with signs of a mild uveitis in some cases.

Adult inclusion conjunctivitis (UNCOMMON) from chlamydial infection is considered as a differential diagnosis here as many of the symptoms and signs are similar to those of adenovirus keratoconjunctivitis, including follicles and a superficial punctate keratitis. A history of a new 'partner' (the organism is sexually transmitted) together with follicles in the upper conjunctival fornix aid the diagnosis. To examine the upper fornix, the upper lid must be double everted using a lid retractor or bimanual cotton-tipped applicators. When in doubt, the tarsal plates are scraped and samples sent to the laboratory for the appropriate investigations.

In children and young teenagers, a specific form of allergic conjunctivitis, *vernal catarrh* (UNCOMMON) leads to photophobia from corneal involvement (see **30** and associated text).

In the more severe form of *erythema multiforme* (Stevens–Johnson syndrome; RARE), acute swelling of the lids is associated with a painful

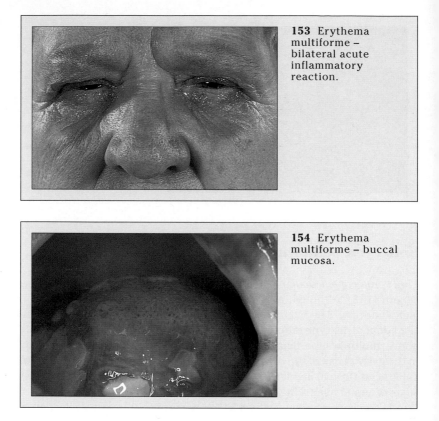

153 Erythema multiforme – bilateral acute inflammatory reaction.

154 Erythema multiforme – buccal mucosa.

membranous conjunctivitis (**153**). Other areas of the body such as the buccal (**154**) and genital mucous membranes may be affected, as well as the skin of the extensor surfaces. The eyes may be the presenting feature. A history of very recent treatment with sulphonamides or other drugs aids the diagnosis.

Arc eye (RARE) characteristically presents 6 hours or more after exposure to an arc-welding flash. With severe sudden onset of pain, lacrimation and photophobia and a typical history the diagnosis is usually straightforward. A bilateral severe punctate staining of the cornea is seen following instillation of local anaesthetic and fluorescein.

Bilateral cases of those conditions outlined under the uniocular section are also considered.

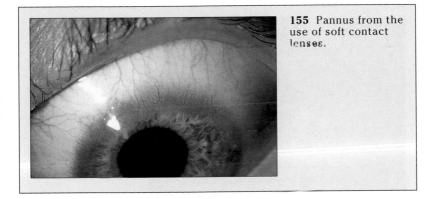

155 Pannus from the use of soft contact lenses.

Red eye(s) following the use of contact lenses

Strategy point
Always use fluorescein to delineate any corneal pathology, as sight-threatening complications must always be excluded. Visual acuity may be 'artificially' reduced due to out-of-date spectacles being worn, or high refractive errors not correcting fully with a pinhole. Contact lens use must not be continued until advised by an ophthalmologist.

Most problems relate to overwear, inadequate cleaning and general care of the lens(es), and sensitivity to the cleaning solutions. Overnight wear is a particularly common basis for problems. Symptoms usually subside on cessation of lens use.

Bacterial conjunctivitis (COMMON) presents as discussed above. Overwear and chipped/dirty lenses leads to sore, diffusely red eyes with punctate keratopathy. Peripheral corneal vascularization may be seen.

Sensitivity to the lens material or cleaning solutions (COMMON) leads to discomfort with itching, excessive mucus and blurring of vision with the lens *in situ*. Multiple papillae are seen on the tarsal plates, the upper tarsae showing giant papillae similar to those seen with vernal catarrh. *Corneal vascularization* with scarring may be seen in some cases (**155**).

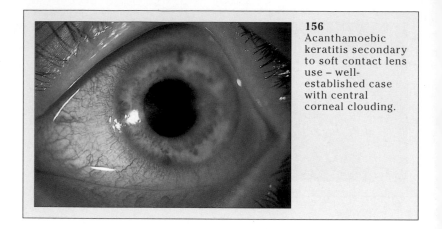

156 Acanthamoebic keratitis secondary to soft contact lens use – well-established case with central corneal clouding.

More rarely, small sterile corneal ulcers, usually peripherally sited, may occur in association with contact lens use. More centrally sited ulcers from bacterial keratitis are generally more painful, require hospitalization and intensive treatment and may progress rapidly with hypopyon/endophthalmitis.

Amoebic keratitis (RARE) produces a painful watery eye with central corneal clouding and an epithelial defect which may be subtle (**156**). The appearance on slit lamp examination is variable – look for enflamed corneal nerves and immune rings in established disease. Disciform keratitis from HSV is the main differential diagnosis.

Red eye following ocular surgery

Strategy point

Find out what the surgery was, when it was performed, and if the patient is still using any topical medications. Complications are RARE following surgery that has been performed by well-trained surgeons using modern microsurgical techniques. However, because of this, it is important to recognize those that do occur.

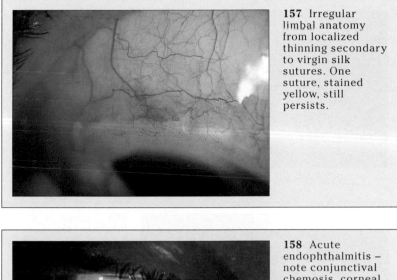

157 Irregular limbal anatomy from localized thinning secondary to virgin silk sutures. One suture, stained yellow, still persists.

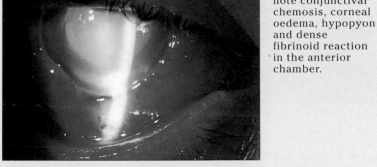

158 Acute endophthalmitis – note conjunctival chemosis, corneal oedema, hypopyon and dense fibrinoid reaction in the anterior chamber.

Cataract surgery

Irritation from *sutures* may occur at any postoperative stage, its nature and timing being dependent on the material used (**157**). Localized redness is seen around the wound site, sometimes with mucus and vascularization of the cornea. Modern sutureless phacoemulsification surgery has reduced this cause of postoperative morbidity significantly. Other complications are rare with modern techniques but may be devastating, as in the case of acute endophthalmitis (**158**). This usually presents within 72 hours of surgery with pain, photophobia, reduced vision, a very injected eye,

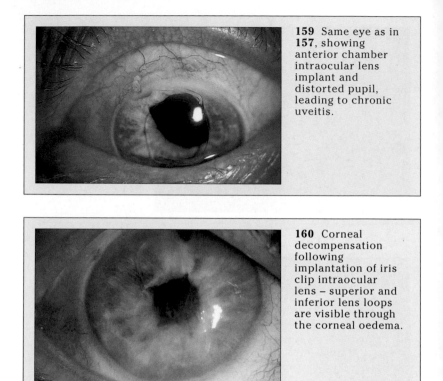

159 Same eye as in **157**, showing anterior chamber intraocular lens implant and distorted pupil, leading to chronic uveitis.

160 Corneal decompensation following implantation of iris clip intraocular lens – superior and inferior lens loops are visible through the corneal oedema.

swollen lids and cloudy media, often with a hypopyon. Early recognition is vital to the eventual outcome.

Chronic uveitis may occur from residual lens matter, sensitivity to lens proteins, or low-grade intraocular infection (**159**). Blurred vision and photophobia may occur and circumlimbal injection with signs of anterior chamber inflammation (KPs, cells and flare). Similar effects can be induced by implant malposition or movement. Cellular deposits on the implant are common and cystoid macular oedema may be detected on fundal examination as the cause of reduced acuity.

Late *corneal decompensation* (**160**) leads to reduced vision, circumlimbal injection and corneal oedema.

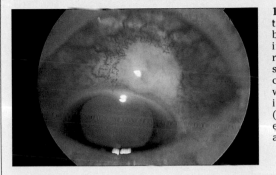

161 Infected trabeculectomy bleb – note the intense inflammatory reaction in the surrounding conjunctiva and pus within the bleb – infection has not (yet) become established in the anterior chamber.

Glaucoma surgery

The presence of a drainage bleb following trabeculectomy may disrupt the tear film and cause irritation, mild stickiness and redness. Other symptoms such as blurred vision and pain suggest *bleb infection* (**161**) and/or endophthalmitis, both rare. The bleb site appears internally turbid or engorged and may demonstrate pus under the conjunctiva in the former. Corneal oedema and hypopyon is added in the latter.

Retinal detachment surgery

Chronic redness of the conjunctiva may occur, often maximal over the site of any explant that has been sutured to the sclera.

Explants sometimes extrude through the conjunctiva, creating irritation and mucus, and may become secondarily infected. A dramatic appearance of an *extruding explant* (**162**) may alarm the patient, and sometimes the attending physician if inexperienced in such matters.

Corneal graft surgery

The most important long-term complication is *graft rejection*. This is usually based on an immunological reaction centred on the corneal endothelium (**163**). It may occur at any time following surgery, although it is most common in the first year. Altered vision, redness and photophobia all may occur and corneal oedema may be seen. Look for new vascularization of the donor, a subtle endothelial rejection line, KPs on the donor but not on the host, and stromal oedema.

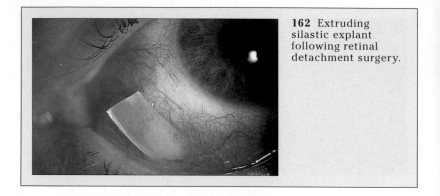

162 Extruding silastic explant following retinal detachment surgery.

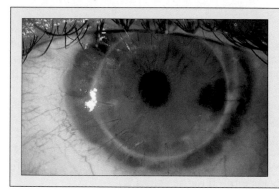

163 Acute corneal graft rejection – note clarity of donor cornea superiorly, and folds in Descemet's membrane and oedema inferiorly.

CHAPTER 7

ABNORMAL LOOKING 'EYE(S)'

Abnormal ocular appearance				
Lids		**Globe**		
Position	*Structure*	*Position*	*Surface*	*Iris/Pupil*
Ptosis	Oedema	Proptosis	Conjunctival	Anisocoria
Entropion	Lesions	Dysthyroid	cysts	Iris tumours
Ectropion	Inflammatory	Enophthalmos	Papilloma	Iris freckles
Retraction	Tumours	Trauma	Melanoma	
			Arcus	

This chapter covers the differential diagnosis of the patient who attends with a primary complaint of an abnormal ocular (or adnexal) appearance. In many cases, such as isolated lid lesions, inspection alone enables the diagnosis, but in others a full history and ocular examination supplemented by special investigations may be necessary.

Strategy point – The History
The chronology of the development of the complaint is important, and any associated symptoms involving vision, pain or other abnormal sensations are sought.

Primary lid abnormalities

These can be divided into abnormalities of position and structure.

Abnormal lid positions
Ptosis – unilateral

Strategy point

In ptosis, the upper eyelid is lower than expected when the patient is looking straight ahead. Remember that the normal upper lid position and contour varies with race. In most white races the lid covers 2 mm of the cornea at 12 o'clock. In any ptosis, exclude coexisting disease of the anterior segment and enophthalmos, both of which may cause a pseudoptosis, check the pupils (Horner's syndrome), and the extraocular movements (IIIrd nerve palsy and myaesthenia).

Congenital ptosis (see **33**) may be secondary to a congenital Horner's syndrome (look for an ipsilateral smaller pupil and paler iris) but is more commonly secondary to a levator dysplasia (an absent upper lid skin crease is a useful sign here). Those associated with other dysmorphic features suggest specific syndromes and are usually bilateral.

Acute unilateral ptosis may be secondary to Horner's syndrome (2 mm ptosis, smaller pupil which reacts normally and perhaps facial anhydrosis), *myaesthenia* (see **120**) (check for fatiguability), *IIIrd nerve palsy* (see **126, 127**) (there may be a subtle ocular movement abnormality with or without pupil dilation) or as a result of *mechanical factors* (**164**) such as chalazion or other local lid disease.

All the above causes are relatively RARE.

Minor degrees of iatrogenic ptosis (COMMON) may occur following intraocular surgery, either due to direct or indirect weakness of the levator which has an insertion into the upper fornix conjunctiva.

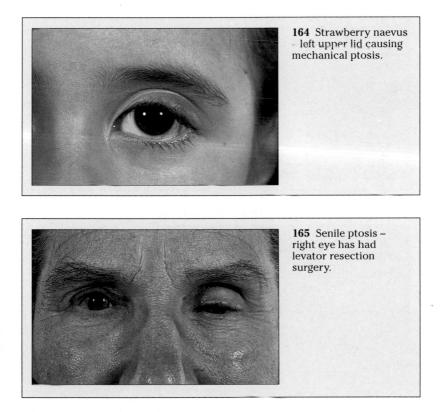

164 Strawberry naevus left upper lid causing mechanical ptosis.

165 Senile ptosis – right eye has had levator resection surgery.

Ptosis – bilateral

Minor degrees of *'senile' ptosis* (**165**) are COMMON and are associated with varying degrees of orbital fat atrophy. Onset is gradual, symmetrical in most cases and lid movements are normal.

Chronic onset bilateral ptosis in a younger age group suggests *myotonic dystrophy* (see **85**) (cataract, male-pattern baldness, featureless expression and 'tonic handshake'), or the rare progressive external ophthalmoplegia (weakness of adduction and later elevation, pigmentary retinopathy in Kearns–Sayre syndrome).

Acute bilateral ptosis is rare and may result from myaesthenia or brain stem disease (**166**).

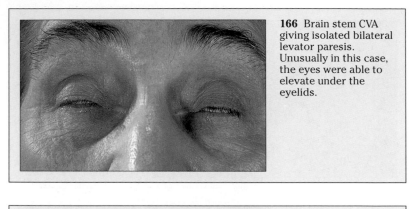

166 Brain stem CVA giving isolated bilateral levator paresis. Unusually in this case, the eyes were able to elevate under the eyelids.

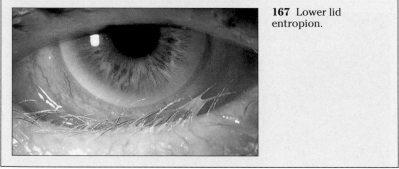

167 Lower lid entropion.

Lower lid positional abnormalities

In 'senile' *entropion* (COMMON), the inverting lid results in lashes abrading the cornea and causing irritation, pain and watering (**167**). The condition may be intermittent in its early stages and a drop of amethocaine 1% often temporarily converts an occult case to an overt one. Abnormal lash position (trichiasis) may induce spasm and secondary entropion, while conjunctival scarring (such as from ocular pemphigoid) causes cicatricial entropion.

In *ectropion* (COMMON) the lid is relatively everted. Subtle medial ectropion results in *epiphora* (see **212–214**), whereas more pronounced ectropion may result in *keratinization* of the tarsal conjunctiva (**168**). Ectropion may be involutional (senile), cicatricial (from tissue loss or contracture), mechanical from lower lid tumours or as a result of neurological disease such as VIIth nerve palsy.

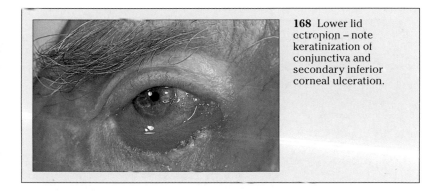

168 Lower lid ectropion – note keratinization of conjunctiva and secondary inferior corneal ulceration.

Lid retraction

More of the globe than usual is visible with lid retraction. It must be differentiated from proptosis which gives a similar appearance, although the two may coexist, particularly in dysthyroid disease.

Lid retraction occurring in the absence of dysthyroid disease is rare.

Abnormal lid structure

Lid oedema (UNCOMMON)

As a result of of the laxity of the tissues, extracellular fluid often gravitates to the lids when no specific local disease is present. Oedema may be positional depending on posture and recumbency and may be transient, resolving when local orthostatic pressures are reduced. For example, a patient in mild right-sided cardiac failure may wake with lid (and local facial) oedema which resolves during the next few hours.

Thyrotoxicosis (see **124**) often results in lid oedema in the acute phase, even in the absence of other ocular signs. Contact allergy, such as from nickel, at sites remote from the eyes may also result in lid oedema and idiosyncratic reactions to drugs may have a similar effect.

Local inflammatory disease of the lid results in oedema with redness and the offending cause must be sought (see below).

Lid lesions

These range from common benign lesions such as chalazia and styes to rarer malignant lesions. In most cases, lesions can be diagnosed by clinical examination alone with a high degree of accuracy, but excision biopsy may be necessary for some atypical lesions. COMMONER lesions are discussed first.

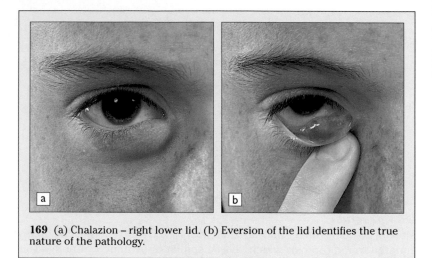

169 (a) Chalazion – right lower lid. (b) Eversion of the lid identifies the true nature of the pathology.

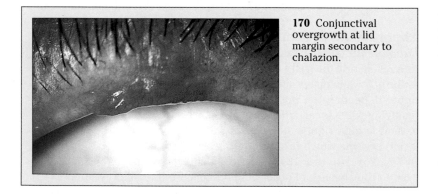

170 Conjunctival overgrowth at lid margin secondary to chalazion.

Chalazion (meibomian cyst or internal hordeolum)

These may present at any age, and as an acute or chronic lesion (**169**). Meibomian gland secretions accumulate focally in the tarsal plate of either the upper or lower lids following occlusion of the gland orifice. Multiple lesions may exist, and *hyperplasia of the conjunctiva* may occur around the meibomian gland orifices (**170**). Acutely infected/inflamed lesions need to be differentiated from styes (look at the internal surface of the tarsal plate)

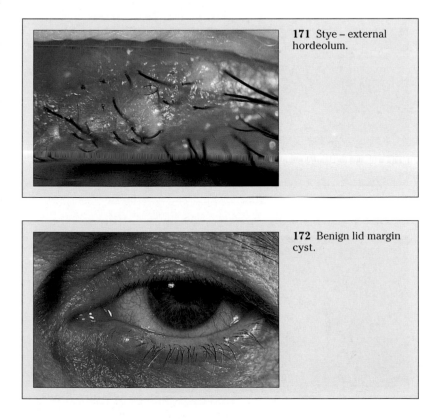

171 Stye – external hordeolum.

172 Benign lid margin cyst.

and chronic lesions from the rare meibomian gland carcinoma (atypical tissue texture at surgery and 'recurrence'). Chronic lesions have a distinctive 'dried pea' texture on palpation.

Stye (external hordeolum)
This is an acute infected lash follicle with a pustular head in the appropriate position (**171**). Again, it may be multiple.

Cysts of Zeis and Moll
These are small, thin-walled cysts near the lid margin containing clear or milky coloured fluid (**172**).

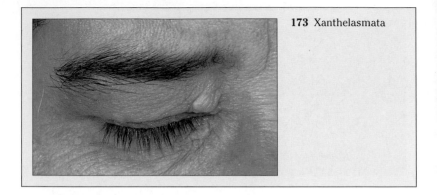

173 Xanthelasmata

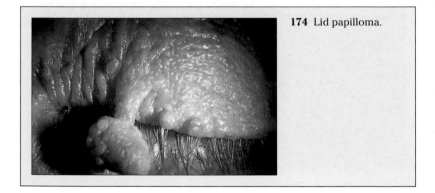

174 Lid papilloma.

Xanthelasmata
These are pale yellow, symmetrical subcutaneous accumulations around the medial lid areas (**173**); they are maximal on the upper lids (check fasting lipids and triglycerides).

Papillomata
These are single or multiple 'wart-like' epithelial growths (**174**).

Solar keratosis
These are focal scaly keratotic lesion(s) in the elderly, and may progress to malignancy.

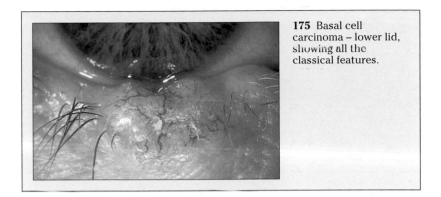

175 Basal cell carcinoma – lower lid, showing all the classical features.

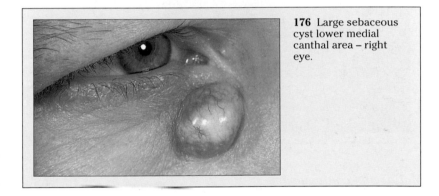

176 Large sebaceous cyst lower medial canthal area – right eye.

Basal cell carcinoma

This is the most common malignant disease of the lids and causes lid notching and loss of lashes when at the lid margin. Classically, it is a locally invasive, nodular, telangiectatic, pearly edged, round or oval lesion with a central depression (**175**). Flatter 'morphoeic' types are less typical.

Sebaceous cyst

This is a slowly growing smooth lesion with a surface punctum and which may become infected (**176, 177**). When in the medial canthal area, it must be differentiated from *acute dacrocystitis* when infected and *mucocele* when not infected (see **132**).

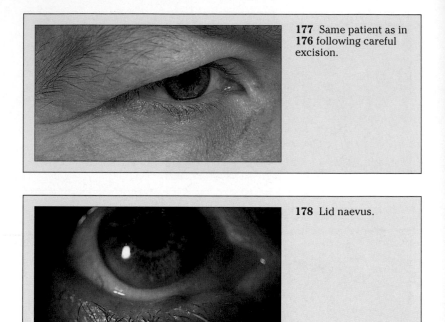

177 Same patient as in **176** following careful excision.

178 Lid naevus.

Molluscum contagiosum
For details, see **133** and associated text.

Pigmented lid naevus
This is a smooth-surfaced, small blue/grey lesion (**178**).

Keratoacanthoma
This is a rapidly growing nodular lesion with a central keratin 'plug' (**179**). Histology may be necessary to differentiate it from a squamous cell carcinoma.

Squamous cell carcinoma
This rare tumour which may develop from Bowen's disease (intraepithelial carcinoma with a red, keratinized, flattish appearance) (**180**). It is locally invasive with the capacity to metastasize – examine the preauricular and cervical lymph nodes. The eccrine cell carcinoma may appear similar (**181**).

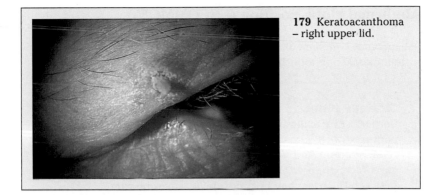

179 Keratoacanthoma – right upper lid.

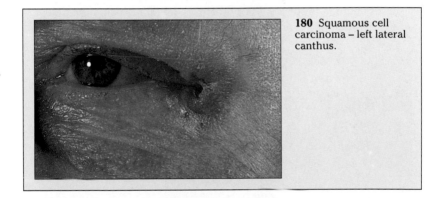

180 Squamous cell carcinoma – left lateral canthus.

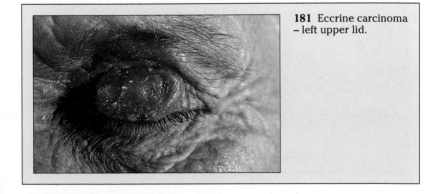

181 Eccrine carcinoma – left upper lid.

Abnormal globe position (UNCOMMON)

Patients may complain of an ocular appearance which is prominent (proptosis) or sunken (enophthalmos).

Strategy point
Care must be taken to ensure that a proptosis in one eye is not confused with an enophthalmos in the fellow eye. Look at the relative upper and lower lid positions in different positions of gaze (see Chapter 2). Remember, up to 2 mm of difference between the eyes may be physiological, and beware facial bone asymmetry. Always perform a full ocular and cranial nerve assessment in proptosis/enophthalmos, including palpation and auscultation of the orbit(s) (**182, 183**).

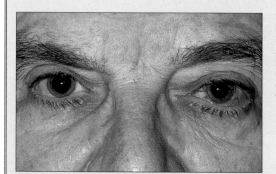

182 Left caroticocavernous sinus fistula with secondary left ptosis – note lower lid position on the left and dilated conjunctival/episcleral vessels.

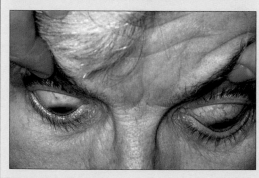

183 Same patient as in **182** viewed from above to demonstrate the left proptosis – the clue from the frontal view was the position of the lower lid on the left.

Proptosis

> **Strategy point**
> Remember to stain the cornea for exposure keratitis in any significant proptosis. Although imaging studies are often employed to determine the diagnosis and/or aid in the management of proptosis, many conditions can be diagnosed by careful detection of physical signs.

Dysthyroid disease is by far the COMMONEST cause of either a unilateral or bilateral proptosis (remember, thyroid function may be normal). Signs of orbital congestion such as conjunctival chemosis and lid oedema may coexist, as may signs of extraocular muscle involvement – restrictive ophthalmopathy (**184**) with discomfort/pain (particularly on upgaze), redness over the rectus insertions and visual dysfunction (reduced acuity, afferent pupil defect, colour vision abnormality, optic disc swelling). Lid retraction and lid lag may occur when the patient is thyrotoxic. The differential diagnosis is usually between pseudotumour and lymphoma if unilateral and lymphoma if bilateral.

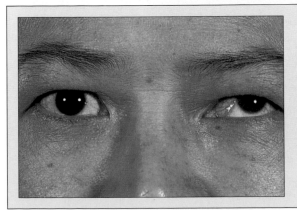

184 Fibrous dysthyroid ophthalmopathy – left eye – giving vertical strabismus secondary to contracture of the left superior rectus.

When unilateral proptosis occurs with acute and severe inflammatory signs, *orbital cellulitis* must be excluded (see **146**).

Chronic proptosis is caused by either an infiltration of orbital tissues such as in dysthyroid disease and 'pseudotumour', benign overgrowth of tissue as in orbital dermoid and capillary haemangioma, malignant expansion as in leukaemia, meningioma of the optic nerve and secondaries, or vascular expansion such as orbital varix and caroticocavernous sinus fistula.

Strategy point

Is the proptosis axial or non-axial? That is, in the primary position, is the globe protruding directly forwards or not?

Axial proptosis results from lesions within the muscle cone; *non-axial proptosis* is a result of extraconal lesions (**185**). The direction of deviation of the globe may help in the diagnosis, e.g. lesions arising from the lacrimal gland result in deviation of the globe downwards and medially.

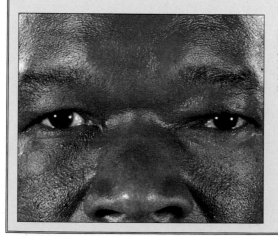

185 Non-axial proptosis – left eye. Left eye is deviated downwards and laterally – proptosis is mild, lesion was in medial wall of orbit.

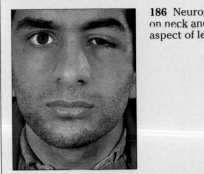

186 Neurofibromatosis with 'café au lait' spot on neck and plexiform neurofibroma in lateral aspect of left upper lid.

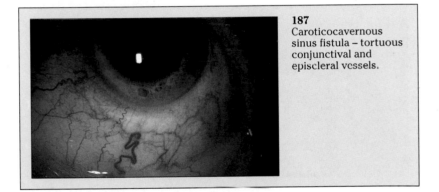

187 Caroticocavernous sinus fistula – tortuous conjunctival and episcleral vessels.

Lesions with characteristic physical signs which cause chronic proptosis of one eye

- *Dysthyroid disease* (see above).
- *Optic nerve gliomas* (young patient with optic atrophy; there may be other signs of neurofibromatosis such as Lisch nodules on the iris and café au lait spots on the skin) (**186**).
- *Dermoid cyst* (palpable smooth lesion usually superior orbit, globe normal; see **34**).
- *Caroticocavernous sinus fistula* (**187**) – slow flow type (middle-aged female with dilated very tortuous veins on the globe surface. There may be secondary raised IOP, transient VIth nerve palsy and orbital bruit. (There may also be blood in Schlemm's canal on gonioscopy, and dilated veins in the retina.)

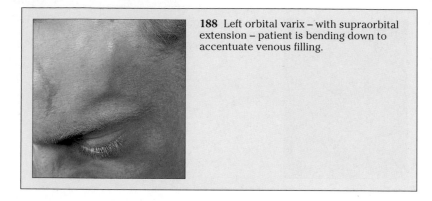

188 Left orbital varix – with supraorbital extension – patient is bending down to accentuate venous filling.

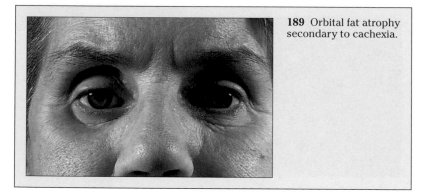

189 Orbital fat atrophy secondary to cachexia.

- *Orbital varix* (**188**). Note the large vein(s) on the conjunctiva or lids. Proptosis increases on Valsalva manoeuvre/bending/compression of the external jugular vein.

Enophthalmos

Bilateral enophthalmos occurs as a result of extreme age and cachexia (**189**). Unilateral enophthalmos is most commonly due to *previous trauma* (see **9**), but secondary tumours and other rare causes are excluded by imaging studies.

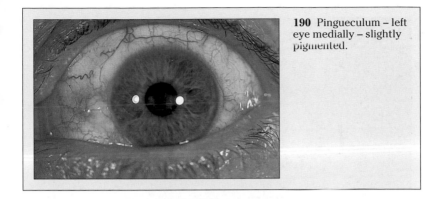

190 Pingueculum – left eye medially – slightly pigmented.

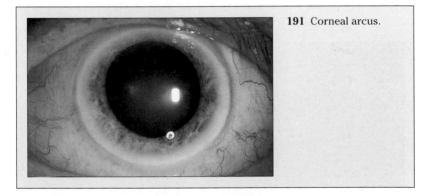

191 Corneal arcus.

Abnormal appearance of the globe

Surface lesions

Surface lesions may cause alarm if they are observed by a third party or in the mirror. Again, COMMONER lesions are described first:

- *Pingueculae* (**190**) are found at the 3 and 9 o'clock positions at the limbus, are slightly raised, and often have a yellowish, irregular surface.
- *Corneal arcus* is a white opacification of the peripheral cornea, with a clear zone before the limbus (**191**). When found in the under 50 age group, check the lipid profile. It is very common in the elderly, but is occasionally noticed by a friend or relative. A unilateral arcus may be associated with a contralateral carotid insufficiency.

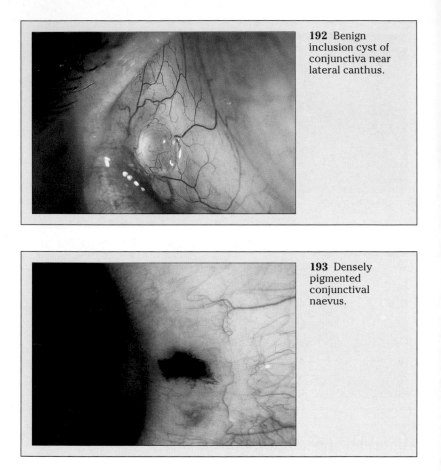

192 Benign inclusion cyst of conjunctiva near lateral canthus.

193 Densely pigmented conjunctival naevus.

- A *pterygium* (see **130**) usually occurs at the medial limbus, growing slowly onto the cornea as a fleshy vascular superficial lesion.
- *Conjunctival cysts* have thin walls containing clear fluid (**192**).
- *Papillomata of the conjunctiva* (see **131**) may arise from the caruncle or elsewhere on the conjunctiva and are raised with a 'stalk'.
- *Benign naevi* are focal, non-ulcerated pigmented areas (**193**). They are more common in blacks.

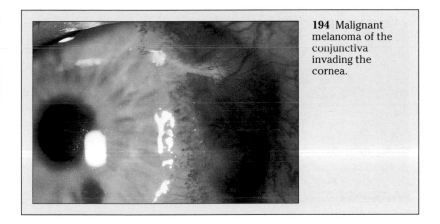

194 Malignant melanoma of the conjunctiva invading the cornea.

- *Malignant melanoma of the conjunctiva* (**194**) may arise from an area of acquired melanosis, often arise at the limbus, and have irregular margins.
- Squamous cell carcinoma of the conjunctiva has an irregular nodular surface and may invade the cornea. Precancerous suspicious lesions are biopsied.

Asymptomatic abnormalities of the iris and pupil

These may also cause concern:

- Physiological anisocoria (a demonstrable difference in pupil size) occurs in up to 25% of normal individuals. Pupil reactions are, of course, normal.
- Anisocoria with otherwise normal reactions occurs in *Horner's syndrome* (see **33**).
- Drug-induced anisocoria is usually due to inadvertent instillation of a dilating agent such as cyclopentolate or atropine. The efferent pupil defect is isolated and does not respond normally to pilocarpine 1% drops (cf. pupil affecting IIIrd nerve palsy).
- *Traumatic mydriasis* with efferent pupil defect occurs commonly after blunt trauma (see **77**).
- *Adie's syndrome*, when acute, results in a dilated pupil which reacts irregularly and slowly to light and accommodative targets (see **113**).

Lesions of the iris may be themselves noticed or may cause pupil

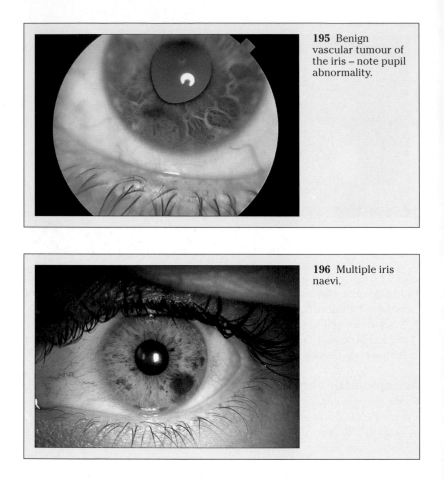

195 Benign vascular tumour of the iris – note pupil abnormality.

196 Multiple iris naevi.

irregularities. Differentiation of benign from malignant lesions may be diffi-cult, the more common lesions being iris freckle, *benign naevus*, *leiomy-oma*, benign cysts, iris atrophy, malignant melanoma and secondary tumours (**195, 196**). (Look for invasion of the angle, ring lesions and 'hidden' lesions with gonioscopy.)

CHAPTER 8

CHRONIC OCULAR UNEASE AND ASSOCIATED HEADACHES

Ocular 'unease'				
Primary symptom				
Aching eyes	*Head/eye ache*	*Sore eye(s)*	*Twitchy eye(s)*	
Refractive	Refractive	Dry eyes	**Lids**	**Eyes**
Muscle balance	Muscle balance	Blepharitis	Stress	Nystagmus
Debility	Debility	Post infective	Dystonia	Superior-
Dry eyes	Dry eyes	Preservatives	Post Bell's	Oblique-
	Drugs	Recurrent abrasion		Myokymia
	Raised ICP	Chronic FB		Stress
	Sinusitis	Trichiasis		
	Cranial arteritis	Entropion		
	Herpes zoster			
		Watery eye(s)		
		Outflow obstruction		
		Irritative disease		
		(Dry eye)		
		Paradoxical tearing		

This chapter covers the differential diagnosis of the patient who attends with chronic eye-related symptoms with no specific visual symptoms.

Strategy point – The History

As physical signs may be few and subtle, a very careful history is vital in the diagnostic process. The patient's lifestyle may play a major role in the symptomatology of chronic ocular discomfort and drug (including self-medication and eyedrop) usage, smoking and alcohol patterns are sought. Previous ocular history must include an optometric history, as many symptoms are related to refractive errors and their correction.

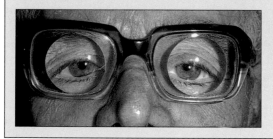

197 Aphakic spectacle-wearing patient (extreme hypermetropia).

'My eyes ache'

A COMMON symptom with many causes, often multifactorial.

Refractive errors and presbyopia are excluded at the outset, particularly when symptoms are related to use of the eyes. Uncorrected astigmatic errors may cause problems when concentrated effort is required such as when reading small print or using a VDU screen. *Hypermetropic patients* (**197**) require a near correction earlier than their emmetropic peers, and although their acuity and reading vision may appear good in short tests in the consulting room, the protracted effort of accommodation gives symptoms of 'eyestrain'. Undercorrected *myopes* (**198**) who narrow their eyes in order to see clearly in the distance are prone to similar symptoms. Overcorrected myopes must accommodate for distance and are rendered 'hypermetropic' by their glasses.

Linked to refractive error is extraocular muscle balance. Strong latent squints (phorias) may cause eye ache due to the effort required to retain

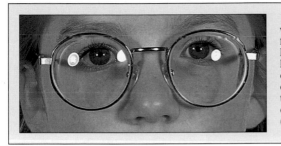

198 Myopic spectacles worn by patient with megalocornea – note how the left spectacle lens 'cuts in' the edge of the hairline near the ear, indicating that these spectacles make objects look smaller (same patient as **27**).

binocular vision. A history of intermittent diplopia, particularly when tired, may be helpful (this is due to a temporary breakdown of the phoria to a manifest squint).

Patients with reduced vision from non-optical causes may also suffer from 'eye ache' in varying degrees of severity. However, it is important to exclude the above causes before attributing symptoms to their primary disease process.

Debility from any cause may induce aching eyes. Systemic viral infections giving a low-grade extraocular muscle myositis induce a dull ache which is worse on moving the eyes or reading. Infections causing chronic disability such as infectious mononucleosis may also be a factor in the symptomatology.

Some patients with *'dry eye' syndrome* (see below) have aching as a predominant symptom, although direct questioning usually reveals other typical symptoms.

'My head and eyes ache'

Although all the causes in the previous section need to be considered here, if headache dominates the picture, additional RARER causes are excluded.

Chronic excess alcohol ingestion may present in this way. Ocular symptoms may be as a result of relative dehydration (red, sore, dry eyes), the residual effect of alcohol and its related toxic by-products (headache, eyeache and vague visual disturbances), or, more rarely, toxic amblyopia (see Chapter 4).

Various prescribed drugs such as nifedipine may induce these symptoms as side effects.

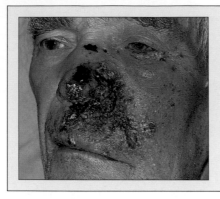

199 Herpes zoster affecting the maxilliary division of the trigeminal.

In raised intracranial pressure from any cause – but particularly from benign intracranial hypertension – chronic headache, usually worse on waking, straining or bending, may be linked with abnormal ocular sensations of 'fullness' or 'aching'. Visual symptoms may be absent, and *papilloedema* is easy to detect in such cases as the disc swelling is usually marked (see **119** and associated text).

Chronic paranasal sinus disease may refer pain to the eyes and the sinus pressure points are tested, although radiographic studies may be necessary to assist in the diagnosis.

Cranial arteritis (see **110**) is excluded in recent-onset headache in the appropriate age group, particularly if symptoms such as pain on chewing or combing/brushing the hair are present. Intermittent vague visual disturbances increase the chance of this diagnosis.

Herpes zoster, in its prodromal phase, may cause severe unilateral pain in and around the eye. A careful search for early skin lesions is made, including posterior to the hair line, and a ipsilateral, diffusely red conjunctiva is common (**199**).

'My eyes feel sore'

Chronically sore, irritable eyes may be the result of a number of external ocular conditions, some of which may also cause more acute symptoms and/or red eyes (see Chapter 6). Discussion here is limited to the scenario when the globes appear relatively normal.

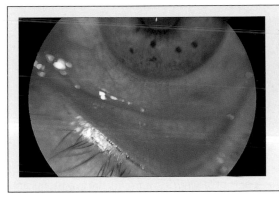

200 Dry eye syndrome with Rose Bengal staining. There is gross staining of the inferior conjunctiva.

Dry eye syndrome (COMMON)

Worthy of a section to itself, dry eye syndrome may cause a multitude of symptoms in different patients. Dramatic descriptions of 'needles in the eyes' and the like are common and do not necessarily relate to the degree of dryness observed or the associated physical signs present in severe disease. The eyes may be described as dry, gritty, sore, burning, aching, tired, painful, or even watery. The last, paradoxical, symptom is as a result of initial drying resulting in reflex tear secretion, and is not uncommon. Associated, and relevant, features of the history may include smoking, regular alcohol ingestion, diuretic or oral contraceptive/HRT usage, or a previous history of chronic lid disease. Symptoms are often brought on by dry heat in the home (gas fires, warm-air central heating), watching TV (low blink rate) and driving with the front screen fan demister on (increased evaporation).

In many cases, other than a subtle reduction in the volume of the tear film which is best seen with the slit lamp before any agent is instilled in the eye, there are no physical signs. In others the 'dry eye' is secondary to meibomian gland dysfunction and obstruction. Blocked ducts may be visible on slit lamp examination. Various tests may be performed, the simplest of which is instillation of *Rose Bengal dye* (**200**). This stains devitalized cells and punctate staining is seen on the lower conjunctiva, rising to involve the lower cornea in more severe cases. The well-known Schirmer's test (in which a bent strip of filter paper is placed in the lower fornix and the accumulation of 'tears' is measured by the wetting rate of the strip) is unreliable unless the eye is grossly dry, particularly if it is used without anaesthetic drops.

In general, when occurring as a result of a well-defined disorder such as

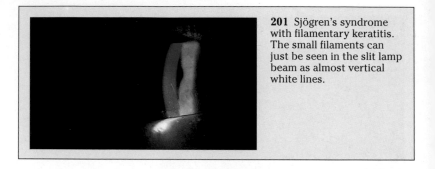

201 Sjögren's syndrome with filamentary keratitis. The small filaments can just be seen in the slit lamp beam as almost vertical white lines.

rheumatoid arthritis and as a part of *Sjögren's syndrome*, the symptoms and signs are more pronounced (**201**). The eyes are very dry, often with mucus in the lower fornix. Filaments of mucus may be seen attached to the corneal epithelium and Rose Bengal stains both these and the adjacent epithelium.

In any case of dry eye syndrome, examine the conjunctiva for signs of subepithelial fibrosis. This may be seen as a result of chronic eyedrop usage, either as a result of the drug or the preservative, or as a sign of *ocular pemphigoid* (**202**). Look for mouth ulceration, often present in pemphigoid.

Do not forget to examine the upper limbus. In *superior limbic keratitis* (**203**), found in isolation and in association with dysthyroid disease, a superior limbitis is seen with superficial punctate keratopathy limited to the superior cornea.

Chronic blepharitis (COMMON)

This may be the primary cause of dry eye symptoms, *marginal ulcers* (see **135**), *styes* and *chalazia* (see **169, 171**). It may also result in a complaint of 'sore eyes' when the patient means 'lids'. Blepharitis can be subdivided into three basic types:

Staphylococcal blepharitis

This occurs following chronic infection of the lid margin with *Staphylococcus aureus* or *Staph. epidermidis* (**204**) The lid margins are red, often with small pustules/stye formation. Loss of lashes may occur, and lid irregularity with notching is common. Very occasionally, other organisms may be involved in immunocompromised individuals (**205**).

Seborrheic blepharitis

This occurs in association with seborrheic dermatitis, particularly of the

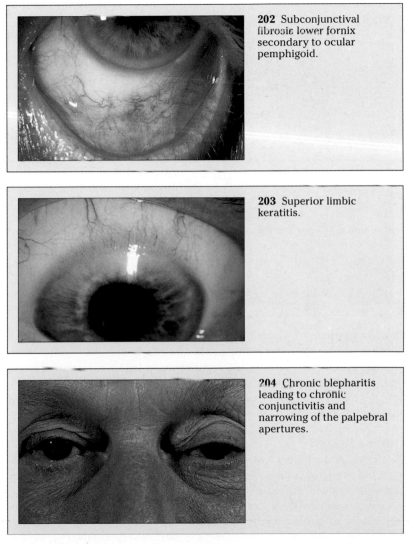

202 Subconjunctival fibrosis lower fornix secondary to ocular pemphigoid.

203 Superior limbic keratitis.

204 Chronic blepharitis leading to chronic conjunctivitis and narrowing of the palpebral apertures.

scalp. The lid margins are not as red, and greasy squames predominate.

A mixed picture is not uncommon, particularly with chronic untreated disease. A superficial punctate keratitis which stains with fluorescein may be seen in all types, usually over the lower cornea.

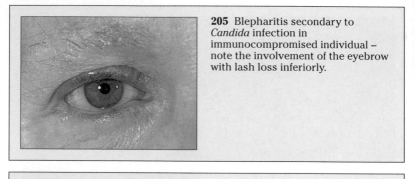

205 Blepharitis secondary to *Candida* infection in immunocompromised individual – note the involvement of the eyebrow with lash loss inferiorly.

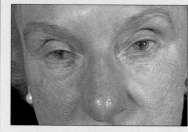

206 Facial rosacea with rhinophyma.

Ocular rosacea

This may occur with or without the other hallmarks of facial rosacea (**206**). Chronic meibomitis leads to lid irregularity and telangiectasia, disturbed tear film and, in more advanced cases, to *corneal thinning* and *opacification/vascularization* (**207**). Corneal melting may occur. A history of facial flushing following the ingestion of small quantities of alcohol is common.

Other causes

Post viral keratoconjunctivitis may linger on for months or years with few signs but symptoms of dry eye syndrome and intermittent blurring that wax and wane. Look for subepithelial focal corneal scarring from adenovirus.

Corneal epithelial dystrophies (RARE) such as Cogan's microcystic dystrophy result in chronic epithelial breakdown often occurring on waking. Symptoms are similar to those of recurrent erosion syndrome (see below) and the eyes are usually white. (Both eyes usually show subtle epithelial microcysts and/or irregular lines in the central zone of the cornea.)

It should not be forgotten that chronic use of any preserved eyedrop or eyewash may cause a chronic toxic keratoconjunctivitis.

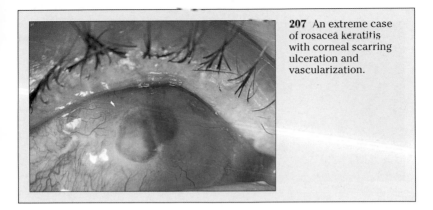

207 An extreme case of rosacea keratitis with corneal scarring ulceration and vascularization.

My eye feels sore

When just one eye is the problem, exclude the following:
* Intermittent *entropion* (see **167**).
* Subtle *ingrowing lash(es)* or a lash extruding from the punctum or caught behind the plica semilunaris (**208**).
* *Chronic foreign body* (**209**).
* *Molluscum contagiosum* (see **133**).
* *Postoperative problems* (see **157–163**).
* *Recurrent erosion/abrasion syndrome.*

The symptoms of this syndrome are characteristic. The patient wakes in the morning or in the night with a sudden pain in their eye, which then waters. The eye may be photophobic. Depending on the severity of the disorder, the symptoms improve as the day goes on, only to return the next morning. Good days may intervene between bad ones. A history of abrasion, often with a child's finger or plant material, is sought. Sometimes the patient may have forgotten the original injury as symptoms may start months after the original trauma.

If examined acutely, the abrasion stains with fluorescein. If seen between attacks, signs may only be visible on slit lamp examination (**210**). (Look for focal areas of irregular epithelium with microcysts within them. Subtle damage to Bowman's membrane may be visible.)

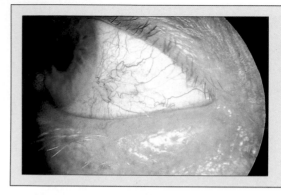

208 Single lower lid lash in aberrant position – the patient only had symptoms on looking to one side when the cornea came into contact with the lash.

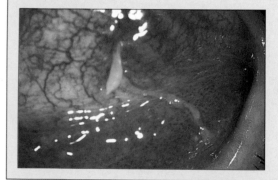

209 Chronic conjunctival reaction secondary to inferior fornicial foreign body. The foreign body has been stained with fluorescein and was adherent to the conjunctiva.

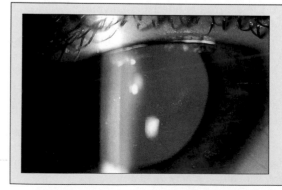

210 Recurrent abrasion syndrome – epithelial microcysts seen by retroillumination (lesions run up to the right from the lower corneal light reflex to the right of the slit beam).

My eye(s) twitches (COMMON)

> **Strategy point**
> One must take care to differentiate between the eyelid that twitches and the eye(s) that twitches.

Lid twitching

Uniocular rapid lid twitching which is intermittent is often a sign of stress in the patient, and resolves when the patient relaxes. Either the upper or lower lid may be involved, with only a small segment twitching.

This must be distinguished from symptoms of the rarer facial dystonia where muscle spasms occur. Severity is variable from intermittent eye lid twitching (usually both lids at once often closing the eye) to hemifacial spasm. Extreme cases are bilateral and incapacitating.

Spasms may occur following recovery from VIIth nerve palsy and lead to a chronically narrowed palpebral aperture.

'Twitching' of the globe(s)

> **Strategy point**
> All twitching eyes are not 'nystagmus'.

Nystagmus is an involuntary, rhythmical oscillation of the eye(s) present in any or all positions of gaze (**211**). Onset of nystagmoid movements must always be taken seriously.

Stress is a COMMON cause of intermittent eye twitching.

In the RARE superior oblique myokymia, a rhythmical uniocular torsional nystagmoid-type movement occurs. It is intermittent and causes uniocular oscillopsia. The 12 o'clock limbal zone of the affected eye rotates rapidly inwards. The history and signs are characteristic and no further investigations are necessary.

Intrusory oscillations (RARE) indicate disease of the midbrain and/or cerebellum. The patient complains of intermittent sudden 'wobbling' of objects from both eyes and a variety of patterns of eye movements may be seen.

211. Nystagmus

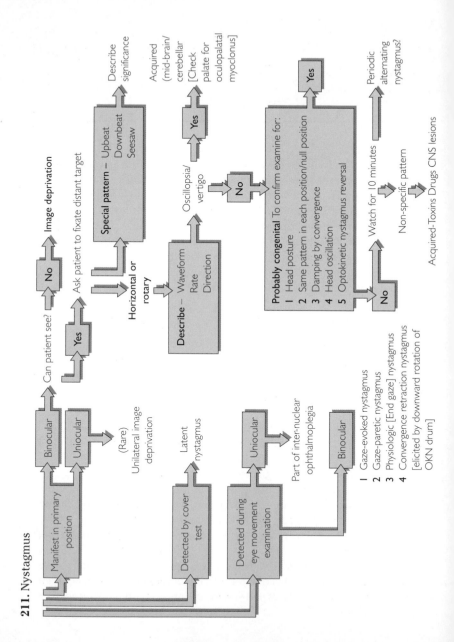

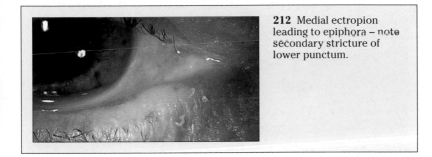

212 Medial ectropion leading to epiphora – note secondary stricture of lower punctum.

Some individuals can induce voluntary nystagmus as a 'party trick'. Occasionally such actions are used, either consciously or unconsciously, in an attempt to achieve financial or other gain. The pattern of the movements (high frequency and low amplitude) and their short duration indicate the diagnosis.

My eye(s) water

In the absence of other symptoms and signs of ocular disease, watering (epiphora) is usually due to restricted lacrimal drainage (COMMON).

> **Strategy point**
> Think anatomically, from the punctum to the nose (see **2**).

Delayed opening of the nasolacrimal duct is discussed in Chapter 3. In adults, epiphora has a number of causes:

- *Medial ectropion* (COMMON) (**212**) – this may be induced by poorly fitting spectacles or be present as a constant feature. It may be as a result of VIIth nerve palsy (neuroparalytic ectropion) (**213**), or as a result of injudicious lid surgery (**214**).
- Punctal occlusion (COMMON) – as 75% of the tears flow through the lower punctum in the normal state, occlusion of this punctum may cause intermittent or occasionally constant epiphora.
- Canalicular occlusion – from various causes, diagnosed by gentle probing with an 00 probe. (A soft stop is found rather than the probe reaching the lacrimal sac and wall of the nose.)

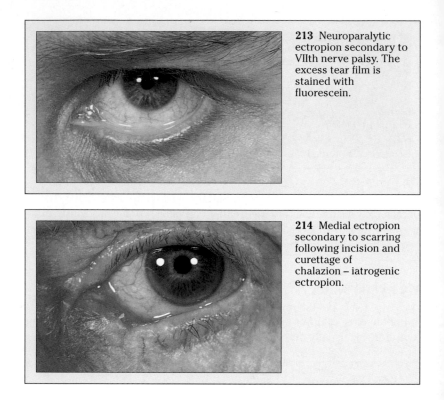

213 Neuroparalytic ectropion secondary to VIIth nerve palsy. The excess tear film is stained with fluorescein.

214 Medial ectropion secondary to scarring following incision and curettage of chalazion – iatrogenic ectropion.

- Nasolacrimal duct obstruction (COMMON) – usually from idiopathic causes but rarely a midline granulomatous lesion (Wegener's) or primary carcinoma. Fluid injected into the lower canaliculus regurgitates via the upper canaliculus. Diagnosis is confirmed with dacryocystography.
- 'Functional blockage' (RELATIVELY UNCOMMON) – it is important to recognize that a system which is patent to syringing may not transfer tears at a normal rate, leading to intermittent epiphora. Diagnosed by lacrimal dacyroscintigraphy where a radiolabelled dye is instilled in the conjunctival sac and its rate of flow to the nose is monitored by a gamma camera.
- Excess lacrimation (COMMON) – reflex tearing is a symptom of many acute and chronic ocular conditions. However paradoxic lacrimation can occur following Bell's palsy due to an aberrant regeneration of the secretory fibres.

CHAPTER 9

OCULAR TRAUMA

Ocular trauma				
Primary symptom				
Blunt	*Sharp*	*Chemical*	*Radiational*	
Periorbital haemorrhage	Lid laceration	Irrigate first	**Acute**	**Chronic**
Subconjunctival haemorrhage	Conjunctival/ corneal abrasion	Measure pH	Thermal	Sunlight
Hyphaema	Conjunctival/ corneal FBs	Particulate matter	Sungazing	Infrared
Iris/lens damage		Alkalis	Arc eye	Iatrogenic
Vitreous haemorrhage	Penetrating injury		Lasers	
Retinal haemorrhage/tear	IOFB		Ionizing	
Choroidal tear				
Ruptured globe				
Blow-out fracture				

Trauma accounts for almost 50% of new attendances at eye casualty departments in the UK. Although most is of a relatively minor nature where full recovery can be expected with simple treatment, it is necessary to distinguish the rarer sight-threatening injuries which need specialist care. Often, the distinction is straightforward, but occasionally injuries which appear relatively benign can progress to blindness.

Those most at risk of ocular trauma are children, young male adults and the elderly. Occupational injuries are rarer in Western society than they were, but still feature prominently in some societies. Sporting- and leisure-related injuries are important causes of visual morbidity in the West. Assaults and war/civil disturbance-related injuries can be devastating.

Injuries can be divided into four basic aetiological categories: blunt, sharp, chemical and radiational. Some injuries may fall into more than one category.

Strategy point – The History

It is tempting to examine the patient immediately as most patients are in distress. However, care with an exact history is important and the story may direct the examiner to seek specific physical signs, or order additional investigations.

In all cases ensure that other injuries and/or medical conditions do not threaten the life of the patient and take the appropriate action. It may be relevant to determine the previous medical history, including hepatitis B, HIV and tetanus status.

Strategy point

The examination – Always attempt to record the visual acuity in both eyes. This may become important later for medical or medicolegal reasons. In many cases, such as corneal abrasions and foreign bodies, simple anterior segment examination with the use of fluorescein dye makes the diagnosis. In others, a full ophthalmological examination is necessary with imaging studies to confirm the full picture.

Blunt trauma

It is often helpful to think anatomically from front to back in blunt trauma to the eye and adnexa, remembering that damage to more posterior structures can occur without severe damage to anterior structures.

Strategy point

Determine the integrity of the globe(s).

Most vulnerable to *rupture* are those eyes which have undergone intraocular procedures, as the sclera/cornea never heals to its original strength

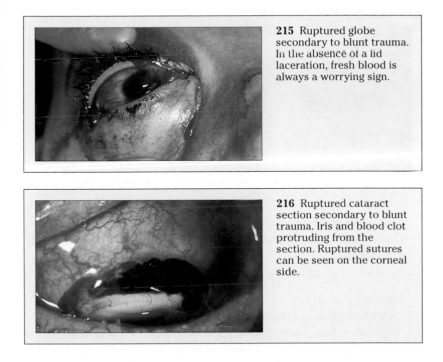

215 Ruptured globe secondary to blunt trauma. In the absence of a lid laceration, fresh blood is always a worrying sign.

216 Ruptured cataract section secondary to blunt trauma. Iris and blood clot protruding from the section. Ruptured sutures can be seen on the corneal side.

following partial or full-thickness penetration. Fresh blood on the surface of the eye with a distorted cornea/iris contour suggests globe disruption and an examination under anaesthetic is necessary (**215, 216**). No further attempt to examine the eye is made as further damage may ensue.

Strategy point

If the globe cannot be examined as a result of severe periorbital haemorrhage, check for the presence of light perception by shining a very bright light through the lids.

Poor or no light perception may indicate coexistent retrobulbar haemorrhage. A proptosis seen clinically or on CT scan increases the risk of optic nerve compression, which requires immediate attention.

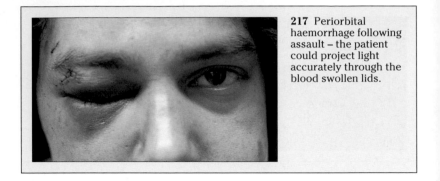

217 Periorbital haemorrhage following assault – the patient could project light accurately through the blood swollen lids.

Most *periorbital haemorrhages* (**217**) resolve spontaneously and detailed examination of the globe can be deferred until an adequate view is possible.

> **Strategy point**
> Any blunt injury sufficient to cause a periorbital haemorrhage or hyphaema may have damaged the posterior segment and/or caused a blow-out fracture of the orbit.

Examine the extraocular movements (blow-out fractures usually reduce elevation + or – depression of the affected eye with pain). There may be a relative enophthalmos and reduced sensation in the area supplied by the infraorbital division of the trigeminal. (CT confirms the diagnosis.)

Check the pupil reactions and proceed to eliminate potential sequelae. An afferent pupil defect indicates extensive retinal damage or, more likely, optic nerve injury.

It is often appropriate to defer detailed fundal examination with pupillary dilation until a hyphaema has cleared, but an undilated assessment of the visible retina is prudent.

Subconjunctival haemorrhage(s) (COMMON) (**218**) may be observed from injury to the conjunctival vessels, as may a *hyphaema* from iris vessel damage (**219**). Look for more severe iris damage. This may take the form of a traumatic *mydriasis* with a dilated pupil, sphincter rupture(s) (see **77**)

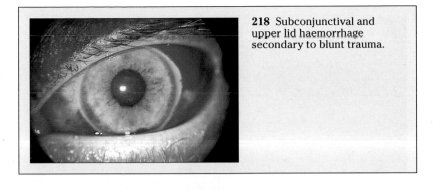

218 Subconjunctival and upper lid haemorrhage secondary to blunt trauma.

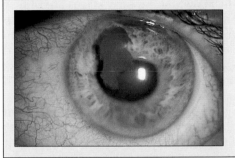

219 Blood clot on superior iris, and small hyphaema secondary to blunt trauma.

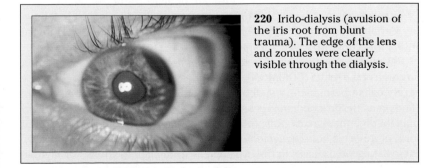

220 Irido-dialysis (avulsion of the iris root from blunt trauma). The edge of the lens and zonules were clearly visible through the dialysis.

and efferent pupil defect, or an *avulsion of the iris root* (**220**). Angle recession involving over 180°, viewable on gonioscopy, increases the chance of raised IOP at a later date.

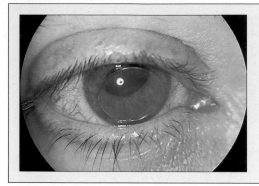

221 Lens subluxation into anterior chamber with secondary glaucoma following blunt trauma. The patient had pre-existing partial subluxation from Marfan's syndrome.

A moderately raised IOP is COMMON in the early stages after blunt trauma. Finding a very low (<4 mmHg) IOP alerts the examiner to the possibility of a posterior scleral rupture. Cyclodialysis may result in protracted hypotony. An over-deep anterior chamber is usually seen and choroidal haemorrhage may be present. CT scanning may help the diagnosis, but exploratory surgery may be necessary to exclude a tear which tends to occur behind the rectus muscle insertions.

Acute cataract (RARE) may follow blunt trauma and there is an increased risk of lens opacity later. *Lens subluxation* (RARE) (**221**) results in iridodonesis and sometimes lenticulodonesis (best seen with the slit lamp on asking the patient to look to either side – damped anteroposterior oscillations of the structures indicate damage to the zonules).

Vitreous haemorrhage (COMMON) in varying degrees is visible following pupillary dilation and prompts careful examination of the peripheral retina for tears or dialysis formation.

Retinal haemorrhages and oedema (*commotio retinae*) may be found in any area of the retina (COMMON) (**222**). Unless they involve the macula, they rarely cause permanent visual loss in themselves. Retinal oedema alone (known as Berlin's oedema) is seen as a pale cream area of the retina and may involve the macula. Resolution occurs but permanent damage in the form of a macula hole or *pigmentary change* may be seen at the fovea (**223**). Pre-existing weaknesses in the eye such as from angioid streaks or myopic degeneration, may result in extensive damage from relatively minor trauma.

Choroidal tears (UNCOMMON) are seen as either arcuate white streaks with or without associated retinal/choroidal haemorrhage (**224**). If the tear transects the fovea, vision is reduced permanently. Severe blunt trauma occurring in the past may result in large areas of *dense choroidoretinal*

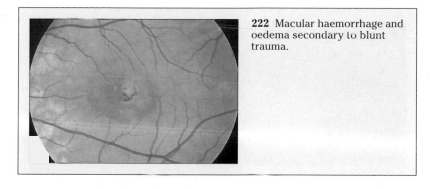

222 Macular haemorrhage and oedema secondary to blunt trauma.

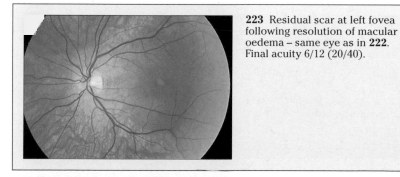

223 Residual scar at left fovea following resolution of macular oedema – same eye as in **222**. Final acuity 6/12 (20/40).

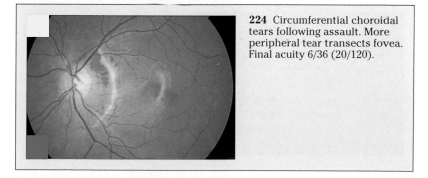

224 Circumferential choroidal tears following assault. More peripheral tear transects fovea. Final acuity 6/36 (20/120).

pigmentation (**225**), with an appearance similar to that seen following inflammatory diseases. *Pre-existing disease of the retina* may render it more vulnerable to trauma (**226**).

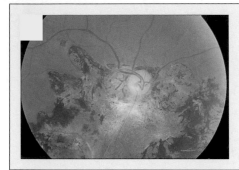

225 Severe chorioretinal scarring following airgun pellet injury – pellet did not penetrate globe and remained in posterior orbit.

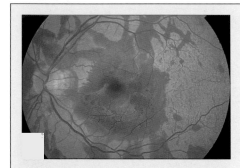

226 Extensive pre-retinal haemorrhage at macula following blunt trauma to a patient with angioid streaks.

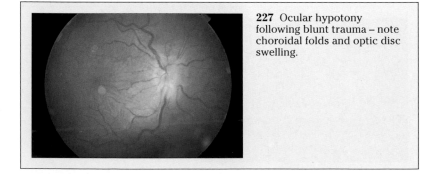

227 Ocular hypotony following blunt trauma – note choroidal folds and optic disc swelling.

Optic disc swelling (RARE) may occur as a result of hypotony or direct injury (**227**). Disc atrophy is a late sign. Very rarely the optic nerve head becomes avulsed with no perception of light.

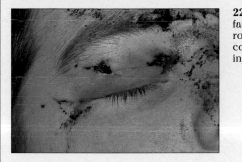

228 Full-thickness lid and facial lacerations following road traffic accident – coexisting penetrating eye injury.

Sharp trauma

Strategy point

If there has been penetration of lid tissue, always exclude the possibility of a retained foreign body, which may be in the orbit. This is particularly true in the case of injuries to children where the history may be unreliable and X-ray, CT or surgical exploration may be necessary.

Eyelid injuries

These are usually plain to see, although some degree of careful cleaning may be necessary to see the full extent of the injury. Tissue is rarely lost except in animal (and human!) bites. Those injuries which involve the medial zone of the lids may involve the lacrimal drainage apparatus and require specialist attention.

Injuries that appear limited to the *eyelid or adnexal tissue* may also have injured the globe (**228**). Always look for subtle signs of ocular penetration (see below).

Injuries to the globe

Minor abrasions of the conjunctiva and cornea (COMMON) are readily diagnosed with the aid of fluorescein (see **11**).

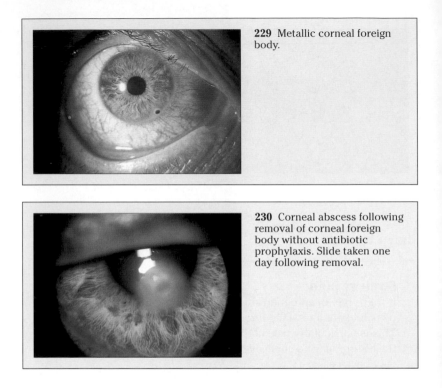

229 Metallic corneal foreign body.

230 Corneal abscess following removal of corneal foreign body without antibiotic prophylaxis. Slide taken one day following removal.

Foreign bodies (FBs) in the conjunctival sac (COMMON) are readily visible inferiorly, but those residing under the upper lid require upper lid eversion. A patient with an *acute subtarsal FB* (see **13**) tends to close the eye because of the corneal pain when opening/closing the eye. Those with a *corneal FB* often delay attending as the irritation increases with time. Metallic FBs are often acquired with grinding instruments or power sanders and a rust ring is commonly seen (**229**).

The importance of instilling a prophylactic antibiotic when removing FBs cannot be overemphasized. Failure to do this risks a *corneal abscess* (**230**).

Penetrating injuries to the globe
These are RARE in most Western societies but may appear in a number of guises (**231–234**), often obvious in severe trauma, but subtle signs are sought:
• Conjunctival laceration, shown with fluorescein, particularly if haemorrhage obscures a clear view of the sclera.

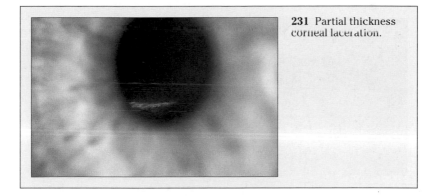

231 Partial thickness corneal laceration.

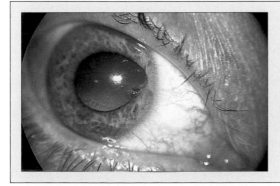

232 Acute penetrating eye injury with pear-drop pupil secondary to road traffic accident. This eye achieved 6/6 (20/20) at the time of photography as the anterior chamber had reformed following iris plugging the corneal wound.

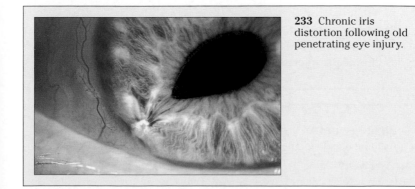

233 Chronic iris distortion following old penetrating eye injury.

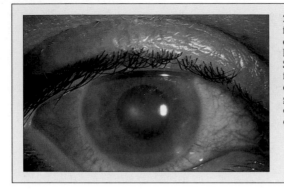

234 Endophthalmitis following penetration of pin into globe at limbus at 4 o'clock. Slide taken 24 hours following injury. Note early corneal abscess, generalized corneal oedema and vitreous opacities.

- An oval *'pear-drop-shaped'* pupil. This probably indicates protrusion of the iris through or up to a corneal laceration and may be seen with a white eye with good vision.
- *Injury to the iris* – often seen as a focal transillumination defect on retroillumination with the slit lamp.
- Lens damage – tears in the anterior and perhaps the posterior lens capsule, best seen with the slit lamp.
- A hazy vitreous – from diffuse haemorrhage or early *endophthalmitis*.
- A soft eye – from leakage of aqueous.
- Protrusion of intraocular contents – iris protruding from the corneal wound can been mistaken for a foreign body!

Strategy point

Any penetrating ocular injury must be admitted for observation as intraocular infection requires prompt management.

Strategy point

Assume an intraocular foreign body to be present in the presence of a suggestive history.

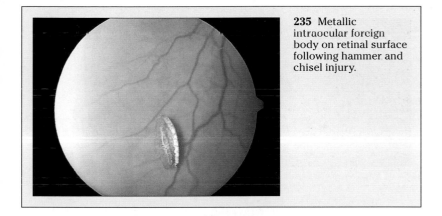

235 Metallic intraocular foreign body on retinal surface following hammer and chisel injury.

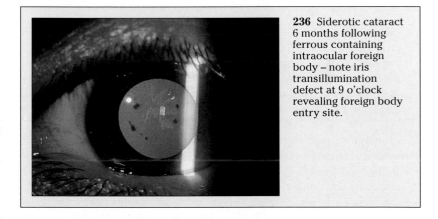

236 Siderotic cataract 6 months following ferrous containing intraocular foreign body – note iris transillumination defect at 9 o'clock revealing foreign body entry site.

Intraocular foreign bodies (IOFBs) (RARE)

These occur most commonly after hammering injuries, particularly with metal-on-metal contact (**235**). The small particles are often self-sterilizing and travel at high speed into the eye, sometimes coming to rest in the orbit or even the brain. Subtle signs of ocular penetration may be seen (see above), or may be missed. An orbital X ray is mandatory even when an apparently normal clinical examination has occurred. Retained iron-containing foreign bodies cause *ocular siderosis* (**236**).

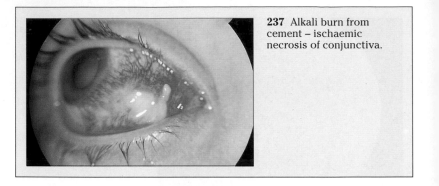

237 Alkali burn from cement – ischaemic necrosis of conjunctiva.

Chemical injuries (COMMON)

Strategy point

In chemical injuries, the initial action is always the same – active irrigation – while a full history is being taken. The irrigation may require instillation of local anaesthetic drops to enable maximal dilution of the noxious agent.

The damage caused to the eye depends on the agent, its volume and concentration, and the time delay to first aid. It is important to identify if particulate matter was involved, as such particles may be very resistant to irrigation and may require removal under general anaesthetic. In general, *alkali injuries* are more severe than acid injuries (**237**), as alkalis penetrate the ocular tissues rapidly. For this reason the finding of a pH above 8 with litmus paper is important.

When irrigation is complete, the eye is stained and the area of corneal epithelial loss observed. Associated signs of severe damage include corneal oedema/opacification and *limbal and/or tarsal ischaemia* (seen as white avascular areas). Raised IOP may be present which may require measurement with non-Goldmann-type tonometers such as the 'tonopen' or a contact pneumatonometer.

Late signs of severe chemical injury include *corneal melting and thinning*, corneal scarring with vascularization, symblepharon, cataract, glaucoma and even corneal perforation (**238**).

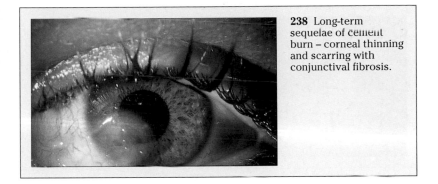

238 Long-term sequelae of cement burn – corneal thinning and scarring with conjunctival fibrosis.

Radiation injuries

The nature of the injury depends on the wavelength, intensity and duration of exposure.

Acute exposure

Acute thermal (infrared) burns are usually limited to the eyelids as a result of the blink reflex (20 ms to closure), although severe injury may result from contact of hot metal or oil with the globe (**239**).

Sungazing, either as a result of psychotropic drugs, mental disease, or in an attempt to view an eclipse can result in foveal burns. In the acute phase a small pale cystic swelling is visible which resolves to produce a foveal scar or cyst/hole. Visual function may recover to a variable degree with time.

Acute ultraviolet burns are as a result of 'arc eye' (COMMON in industrial zones) (see Chapter 6). Snow blindness is of similar aetiology despite the longer exposure. Loss of corneal epithelium is seen in severe cases and photophobia and lacrimation is profound. Occasionally, overexposure to the radiation from a sunlamp or sunbed induces facial burns. Protective goggles usually result in no ocular involvement.

Acute exposure to laser energy of a wavelength which reaches the retina may result in foveal damage similar to that produced by sungazing.

Acute exposure to high doses of ionizing radiation may cause signs of acute anterior segment inflammation with chronic keratitis, cataract and retinal/optic nerve damage occurring at any time after 6 months if the individual survives.

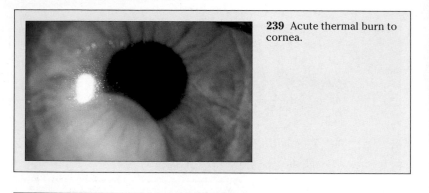

239 Acute thermal burn to cornea.

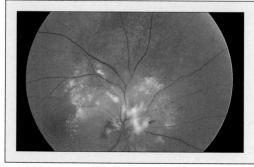

240 Radiation retinopathy following cobalt beam irradiation to malignant melanoma. Small vessels of the optic nerve have also been involved resulting in optic nerve infarction.

Chronic exposure (RARE)

Chronic exposure to sunlight is associated with pengueculae and pterygia, actinic keratosis of the skin, malignant melanoma and perhaps cataract in susceptible individuals.

Long-term exposure to infrared irradiation may very rarely lead to exfoliative cataract and is occasionally seen in unprotected glassblowers or furnace workers.

Iatrogenic disease as a result of fractionated doses of radiotherapy or plaque therapy for ocular tumours may cause a variety of ocular problems depending on the dosage that each part of the eye has received. Dry eyes are common, as is cataract (most sensitive ocular structure) followed by the retinal capillaries and the optic nerve. *Radiation retinopathy* (**240**) usually occurs after a latent period of 18 months or so and telangiectatic vessels with haemorrhages, oedema and hard exudates are seen, usually in the macular area.

CHAPTER 10

OPHTHALMOLOGY THROUGHOUT THE WORLD

Global ophthalmology		
Chronic visual loss	**Acute ocular symptoms**	**Incidental findings**
Cataract	Trachoma	Schistosomiasis
Trachoma	Loa Loa	
Vitamin A deficiency	Cysticercosis	
Glaucoma	Ocular myiasis	
Leprosy		
Diabetic retinopathy		
Onchocerciasis		

Patterns of eye disease and their modes of presentation vary in different locations as a result of the manner in which humans interact with their environment; a number of factors may be involved which often interact:

- Geographical location influences the infectious agents that are endemic.
- Genetic susceptibility to certain eye conditions, e.g. glaucoma is much more common in certain races, and the type may also vary – chronic angle closure in the East and pseudoexfoliative in Scandinavians, Greeks and certain African tribes. Rhegmatogenous retinal detachment is rare in blacks, as is age-related macular degeneration.
- Local living conditions – poverty is linked with malnutrition, poor hygiene, lack of fresh water and the prevalence of other coexistent disease.
- Religious or other beliefs – may lead to a mistrust of medical care with a fear of hospitals and late presentation.
- Lack of access to medical care (**241**).
- Local conditions of work – may put individuals at increased risk of occupational eye disease, particularly trauma.
- Political priorities influence much of the above.

The availability, cost and speed of modern air travel increases the importance of a knowledge of ocular conditions not usually found in the examiner's area.

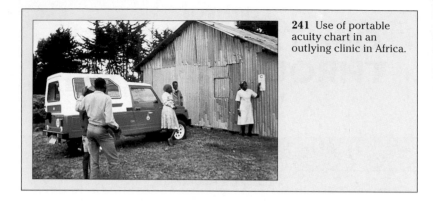

241 Use of portable acuity chart in an outlying clinic in Africa.

Causes of chronic visual loss

Diseases which are found in Western societies also cause significant morbidity in other countries. History and clinical examination are similar to those described in Chapter 4, although later presentation is often the norm.

Cataract has overtaken other tropical diseases as the major cause of blindness world-wide (**242**). Cataract occurs at a younger age in some societies and this has been linked to malnutrition, severe diarrhoea, excess exposure to sunlight and genetic susceptibility among others.

Glaucoma tends to present symptomatically and therefore at a late stage where opportunistic screening is not performed (**243**).

Diabetic retinopathy is a particular problem in those from the Indian subcontinent because of the increased prevalence of Type II diabetes and recent improvements in health care resulting in a longer life span.

Other causes of chronic visual loss are found in appropriate geographical areas, the most common of which are discussed below.

Vitamin A deficiency

This is mainly a disease of children in areas where the diet is deficient in green vegetables and fish. In Indonesia, it has been found that the most effective way to screen for subclinical disease is to ask the mother if the child has any problems in dim light. Thus, nyctalopia precedes the anterior segment manifestations.

In a suspect, examine the conjunctiva for *xerosis* (**244**), an irregular rippling of the conjunctival surface as a result of keratinization, and *Bitot's*

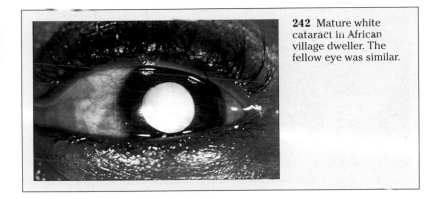

242 Mature white cataract In African village dweller. The fellow eye was similar.

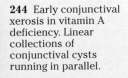

243 Intraocular pressure measurement with the portable battery-operated Perkins tonometer.

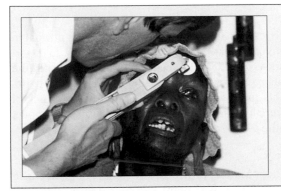

244 Early conjunctival xerosis in vitamin A deficiency. Linear collections of conjunctival cysts running in parallel.

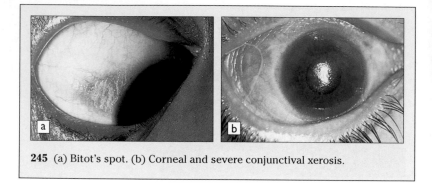

245 (a) Bitot's spot. (b) Corneal and severe conjunctival xerosis.

spot (**245a**), foamy, white lesions at the limbus. Visual acuity is normal in the absence of corneal involvement.

Corneal xerosis appears as irregular thickened epithelium and heralds the onset of keratomalacia where central corneal melting with the risk of perforation occurs (**245b**). This process may be precipitated by an attack of measles, and is more severe if protein deficiency coexists. Herpes simplex infection may complicate the picture and must be considered in a severe case.

Trachoma

Corneal scarring from trachoma was previously the most common cause of blindness world-wide before it was displaced by cataract. Cases of established disease are seen in those who are visiting or who have settled in the West, with variable visual loss. Improvements in public health in the West now mean that it is mainly a disease of subtropical and tropical climes, being mainly found in Africa, the Middle East and Asia. Recurrent infection is required for the chronic sight-threatening disease.

Vascularized corneal scars, usually maximal superiorly, are seen in association with entropion of the upper or occasionally the lower lids which occurs as a result of a *cicatrizing of the tarsal plates*, observable as transversely orientated gliotic tissue (**246**). Herbert's pits indicate the sites of previous limbal follicles and are seen as focal thinned areas of peripheral cornea, usually seen at the upper limbus.

The eye(s) may be dry as a result of poor tear secretion, or watery from irritation combined with occlusion of the lacrimal drainage system.

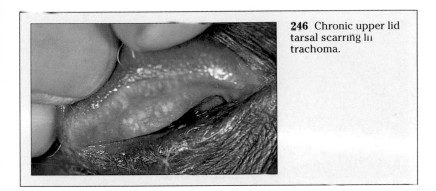

246 Chronic upper lid tarsal scarring in trachoma.

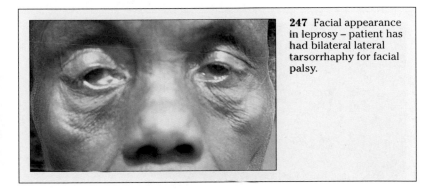

247 Facial appearance in leprosy – patient has had bilateral lateral tarsorrhaphy for facial palsy.

Leprosy

Very rarely seen in the West, this disorder is common in more temperate parts of South America and the Far East.

Chronic loss of vision is as a result of corneal scarring, chronic uveitis and cataract, secondary glaucoma or a combination of these.

The *typical facial features* of the disease, namely loss of the bridge of the nose, loss of the lateral portions of the eyebrows, VIIth nerve palsy, and thickening of the facial skin suggest the diagnosis if it is not already known (**247**). Ocular features include madarosis (loss of the eyelashes and eyebrows), lower lid ectropion, corneal scarring, sometimes with ghost vessels, corneal anaesthesia, thickened corneal nerves, signs of a low-grade uveitis and/or scleritis and small pupils. Secondary infection with ulceration is common. Visual field defects from glaucoma may be demonstrated.

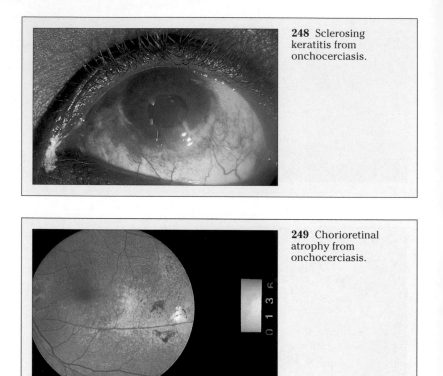

248 Sclerosing keratitis from onchocerciasis.

249 Chorioretinal atrophy from onchocerciasis.

Onchocerciasis

Seen in parts of Central America and Africa where both the filarial worm and its vector, the Black fly, are endemic, this condition is known as 'river blindness'.

Visual loss is as a result of *chronic keratitis* (**248**), uveitis, cataract, secondary glaucoma and, rarely, optic neuritis.

Live microfilaria may be observed in the anterior chamber with a coexistent conjunctivitis. If posterior synechiae and cataract are sufficiently limited to allow a view of the fundus, *pigment clumping temporal to the macula* may be seen (**249**).

Subcutaneous nodules elsewhere in the body can be aspirated in a search for microfilaria, or a conjunctival biopsy may be of assistance in dubious cases.

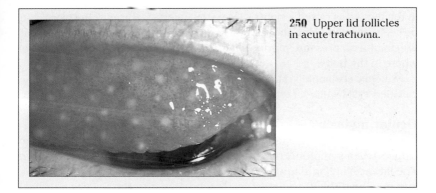

250 Upper lid follicles in acute trachoma.

Causes of acute ocular symptoms

In addition to those conditions described in previous chapters, certain conditions outlined below require special mention in a global context.

Trachoma
The acute stages of this infection with *Chlamydia trachomatis* present as a bilateral mucopurulent conjunctivitis. Follicles are seen in the conjunctival fornices, the upper tarsal plate and the limbus (**250**). A superficial punctate keratopathy may be present. Like most causes of infective conjunctivitis it is self-limiting, but recurrent infection leads to the chronic disease (see above).

Loa Loa
This disorder, found in Africa, may cause ocular problems from the migration of the worm into the orbit where it may appear under the conjunctiva, giving symptoms of 'something moving in my eye' or pain. More rarely, the worm may migrate into the anterior chamber, the vitreous or the retina where it can be observed as a motile body.

Cysticercosis
Caused by ingestion of the active worm *Taenia solium* in undercooked pork, the ocular manifestations of the disease, which is usually found in the tropics and subtropics, tend to involve the retina and choroid. Vision is disturbed by the physical presence of the worm(s) which can be visualized

in the fundus as raised lesion(s). Occasionally the features of the worm can be seen, its head being about 1 mm in diameter. Subconjunctival cysts that are painful on pressure may be seen. Subcutaneous cysts are sought elsewhere in the body.

Systemic eosinophilia is a constant feature. Imaging of the brain may show calcified cysts while X rays of the limbs often show similar calcification.

Ocular myiasis

Acute conjunctival infestation with the larvae of flies is considered in the tropics when symptoms of severe itching, burning and lacrimation occur. The larvae, similar in appearance to maggots, congregate in the fornices and may be difficult to detect as they burrow into the tissues. Surgical exploration may be necessary if doubt exists, the larvae being paralysed by cocaine 10% drops.

Incidental ocular findings

Schistosomiasis is endemic in Egypt and certain areas of Asia. While it causes little in the way of symptoms, the conjunctival nodules may suggest other diagnoses such as tuberculosis or sarcoidosis. Diagnosis is by microscopic examination of biopsy material with the bilharzial ova at the centre of a granulomatous reaction.

GLOSSARY

Accommodation – the process by which the eye changes focus from a distant to a near object.

Amaurosis fugax – a temporary loss of vision with full recovery.

AMPPE – acute multifocal placoid pigment epitheliopathy.

Anisocoria – where there is a demonstrable difference in pupil size.

Anisometropia – a condition when there is a significant difference in the refractive error between the two eyes.

Aphakia – without a lens.

ARMD – age-related macular degeneration.

Astigmatism – an optical error, usually arising in the cornea, in which light rays are brought to more than one focus.

Bell's phenomenon – where the eye elevates upon forced closure of the lids – a protective mechanism.

CF – Count Fingers, a level of vision in an eye, usually expressed at a certain distance, e.g. CF at 1 m. Indicates better vision than HM (see below).

Choriocapillaris – the rich bed of capillaries in the choroid which supplies the photoreceptor layer of the retina with nutrients.

CMV – cytomegalovirus.

Coloboma – a congenital absence of part of an ocular tissue.

CRVO – central retinal vein occlusion.

CSG – chronic simple glaucoma.

CVA – cerebrovascular accident.

Cyclodialysis – a cleft between the ciliary body and sclera.

Cycloplegia – drug-induced paralysis of the ciliary muscle. Used to obtain an objective refraction in children.

Dendrite – a pattern of corneal ulceration (looking like the branches of a tree), usually as a result of herpes simplex virus infection.

Diplopia – double vision, may be monocular (one eye) or binocular (only present with both eyes open).

Dioptre – a measure of lens strength, the reciprocal of the focal length in metres.

Electroretinogram – a diagnostic test in which the electrical response of the retina is measured.

Endophthalmitis – global intraocular inflammation, usually infective.

Epicanthus – a fold of skin, found in young children, which may cover the medial aspect of the lids.

Follicle – a germinal centre in the conjunctiva, usually multiple in the lower and/or upper fornix. Appears as a raised pink mound with a paler centre.

Gaze palsy – where the eyes cannot look in one direction.

Hemianopia – a loss of visual field in both eyes.

HM – hand movements, a level of vision in an eye.

Homonomous – in a similar position in space, when related to field defects.

Hypermetropia – long-sightedness, parallel light rays will focus beyond the retina if the eye is in a relaxed state of accommodation.

Hyphaema – a fluid level of blood in the anterior chamber.

Hypopyon – a fluid level of white cells in the anterior chamber.

Hypotony – a very low intraocular pressure.

HSV – herpes simplex virus.

ICP – intracranial pressure.

Iridodonesis – abnormal oscillations of the iris found when the usual support from the natural lens is altered or lost.

Keratic precipitates (KPs) – accumulations of white cells on the corneal endothelium.

Keratitis – inflammation of the cornea.

Lenticulodonesis – abnormal oscillations of the lens following zonule rupture.

LP – Light perception.

Limbus – the junctional zone between the cornea and the sclera.

Micropsia – when the image of an object is perceived smaller than normal, usually as a result of macular pathology.

MRI – magnetic resonance imaging.

Meiosis – constriction of the pupil.

Myopia – short-sightedness, parallel light rays (from a distant object) are brought to a focus in front of the retina.

NLP – no light perception.

Nystagmus – a rhythmical oscillation of the eyes.

Optokinetic drum – a rotating cylinder with alternating black and white stripes. Used for inducing eye movements.

Papillitis – inflammation of the optic nerve head.

Papilloedema – a swollen optic nerve head as a result of raised intra-cranial pressure.

Photophobia – an inability to tolerate bright lights.

Pigment epithelium – a monolayer of cells between the retina and the choroid, important to retinal function.

Punctate keratopathy – or SPK, a corneal epithelial sign with multiple epithelial erosions, dot-like staining.

RAPD – relative afferent pupil defect.

Refraction – the process by which an optical error is determined (in pure optics – the deviation which is induced when light moves from one medium to another of different density).

Scotoma – a pathological defect in the visual field of one eye.

Synechiae – adhesions between the iris and other structures, posterior synechiae are to the lens, anterior to the cornea.

Tonometer – device that measures IOP.

Uveitis – inflammation of the uveal tract, the vascular coat of the eye.

Webino – 'Wall-eyed' bilateral internuclear ophthalmoplegia.

INDEX